PENGUIN MODERN CLASSICS

Illness as Metaphor and AIDS and Its Metaphors

Susan Sontag was born in Manhattan in 1933 and studied at the universities of Chicago, Harvard and Oxford. She is the author of four novels, *The Benefactor*, *Death Kit*, *The Volcano Lover* and *In America*, which won the 2000 National Book Award for fiction; a collection of stories, *I, etcetera*; several plays, including *Alice in Bed*; and six books of essays, among them *Illness as Metaphor* and *AIDS and Its metaphors*, and *Regarding the Pain of Others*, which are published by Penguin. Her books are translated into thirty-two languages. In 2001 she was awarded the Jerusalem Prize for her body of work, and in 2003 she received the Prince of Asturias Prize for Literature and the Peace Prize of the German Book Trade. She died in December 2004.

SUSAN SONTAG

Illness as Metaphor and
AIDS and Its Metaphors

PENGUIN BOOKS

PENGUIN CLASSICS

Published by the Penguin Group
Penguin Books Ltd, 80 Strand, London WC2R ORL, England
Penguin Group (USA) Inc., 375 Hudson Street, New York, New York 10014, USA
Penguin Group (Canada), 90 Eglinton Avenue East, Suite 700, Toronto, Ontario, Canada M4P 2Y3
(a division of Pearson Penguin Canada Inc.)
Penguin Ireland, 25 St Stephen's Green, Dublin 2, Ireland, (a division of Penguin Books Ltd)
Penguin Group (Australia), 250 Camberwell Road, Camberwell, Victoria 3124, Australia
(a division of Pearson Australia Group Pty Ltd)
Penguin Books India Pvt Ltd, 11 Community Centre, Panchsheel Park, New Delhi – 110 017, India
Penguin Group (NZ), 67 Apollo Drive, Rosedale, North Shore 0632, New Zealand
(a division of Pearson New Zealand Ltd)
Penguin Books (South Africa) (Pty) Ltd, 24 Sturdee Avenue, Rosebank, Johannesburg 2196, South Africa

Penguin Books Ltd, Registered Offices: 80 Strand, London WC2R ORL, England

www.penguin.com

Illness as Metaphor first published in the USA by Farrar, Straus & Giroux 1978
Published in Great Britain by Allen Lane 1979
Published in Penguin Books 1983

AIDS and its Metaphors first published in the USA by Farrar, Straus & Giroux 1989
Published simultaneously in Canada by Collins Publishers, Toronto
Published in Great Britain by Allen Lane 1989
Published in Penguin Books 1990

Illness as Metaphor and *AIDS and Its Metaphors* published together in one volume in Penguin Books 1991
Reprinted in Penguin Classics 2002

023

Illness as Metaphor copyright © Susan Sontag, 1977, 1978
AIDS and Its Metaphors copyright © Susan Sontag, 1988, 1989
This volume copyright © Susan Sontag, 1991
All rights reserved

The moral right of the author has been asserted

Illness as Metaphor appeared in an earlier version in *The New York Review of Books*, Vol. xxiv,
Nos 21 and 22 (26 January 1978); Vol. xxv, No. 1 (9 February 1978); Vol. xxv, No. 2 (23 February 1978).
The lines from 'Miss Gee' on pp. 49–50 are from *Collected Poems* by W. H. Auden, edited by Edward
Mendelson, copyright 1940 and renewed 1968 by W. H. Auden; reprinted by permission of
Random House, Inc. Quotations from Karel Čapek's *The White Plague* are from the translation by
Michael Henry Heim, published in *Cross Currents*, 7 (1988)

Printed in England by Clays Ltd, St Ives plc

978-0-141-18712-9

www.greenpenguin.co.uk

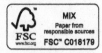

Contents

ILLNESS AS METAPHOR

Illness is the night-side of life, a more onerous citizenship. Everyone who is born holds dual citizenship, in the kingdom of the well and in the kingdom of the sick. Although we all prefer to use only the good passport, sooner or later each of us is obliged, at least for a spell, to identify ourselves as citizens of that other place.

I want to describe, not what it is really like to emigrate to the kingdom of the ill and live there, but the punitive or sentimental fantasies concocted about that situation: not real geography, but stereotypes of national character. My subject is not physical illness itself but the uses of illness as a figure or metaphor. My point is that illness is *not* a metaphor, and that the most truthful way of regarding illness – and the healthiest way of being ill – is one most purified of, most resistant to, metaphoric thinking. Yet it is hardly possible to take up one's residence in the kingdom of the ill unprejudiced by the lurid metaphors with which it has been landscaped. It is toward an elucidation of those metaphors, and a liberation from them, that I dedicate this inquiry.

Chapter One

Two diseases have been spectacularly, and similarly, encumbered by the trappings of metaphor: tuberculosis and cancer.

The fantasies inspired by TB in the last century, by cancer now, are responses to a disease thought to be intractable and capricious – that is, a disease not understood – in an era in which medicine's central premise is that all diseases can be cured. Such a disease is, by definition, mysterious. For as long as its cause was not understood and the ministrations of doctors remained so ineffective, TB was thought to be an insidious, implacable theft of a life. Now it is cancer's turn to be the disease that doesn't knock before it enters, cancer fills the role of an illness experienced as a ruthless, secret invasion – a role it will keep until, one day, its etiology becomes as clear and its treatment as effective as those of TB have become.

Although the way in which disease mystifies is set

against a backdrop of new expectations, the disease itself (once TB, cancer today) arouses thoroughly old-fashioned kinds of dread. Any disease that is treated as a mystery and acutely enough feared will be felt to be morally, if not literally, contagious. Thus, a surprisingly large number of people with cancer find themselves being shunned by relatives and friends and are the object of practices of decontamination by members of their household, as if cancer, like TB, were an infectious disease. Contact with someone afflicted with a disease regarded as a mysterious malevolency inevitably feels like a trespass; worse, like the violation of a taboo. The very names of such diseases are felt to have a magic power. In Stendhal's *Armance* (1827), the hero's mother refuses to say 'tuberculosis,' for fear that pronouncing the word will hasten the course of her son's malady. And Karl Menninger has observed (in *The Vital Balance*) that 'the very word "cancer" is said to kill some patients who would not have succumbed (so quickly) to the malignancy from which they suffer.' This observation is offered in support of anti-intellectual pieties and a facile compassion all too triumphant in contemporary medicine and psychiatry. 'Patients who consult us because of their suffering and their distress and their disability,' he continues, 'have every right to resent being plastered with a damning index tab.' Dr. Menninger recommends that physicians generally abandon 'names' and 'labels' ('our function is to help these people, not to further afflict them') – which would mean, in effect, increasing secretiveness and medical paternalism. It is not naming as such that is pejorative or damning, but the name 'cancer.' As long as a particular disease is treated as an evil, invincible predator, not just a disease, most people with cancer will indeed be demoralized by learning what disease they have. The solution is hardly to stop telling cancer patients the truth, but to rectify the conception of the disease, to de-mythicize it.

When, not so many decades ago, learning that one had TB was tantamount to hearing a sentence of death – as today, in the popular imagination, cancer equals death – it was common to conceal the identity of their disease from tuberculars and, after they died, from their children. Even with patients informed about their disease, doctors and family were reluctant to talk freely. 'Verbally I don't learn anything definite,' Kafka wrote to a friend in April 1924 from the sanatorium where he died two months later, 'since in discussing tuberculosis ... everybody drops into a shy, evasive, glassy-eyed manner of speech.' Conventions of concealment with cancer are even more strenuous. In France and Italy it is still the rule for doctors to communicate a cancer diagnosis to the patient's family but not to the patient; doctors consider that the truth will be intolerable to all but exceptionally mature and intelligent patients. (A leading French oncologist has told me that fewer than a tenth of his patients know they have cancer.) In America – in part because of the doctors' fear of malpractice suits – there is now much more candor with patients, but the country's largest cancer hospital mails routine communications and bills to outpatients in envelopes that do not reveal the sender, on the assumption that the illness may be a secret from their families. Since getting cancer can be a scandal that jeopardizes one's love life, one's chance of promotion, even one's job, patients who know what they have tend to be extremely prudish, if not outright secretive, about their disease. And a federal law, the 1966 Freedom of Information Act, cites 'treatment for cancer' in a clause exempting from disclosure matters whose disclosure 'would be an unwarranted invasion of personal privacy.' It is the only disease mentioned.

All this lying to and by cancer patients is a measure of how much harder it has become in advanced industrial societies to come to terms with death. As death is now an offensively meaningless event, so that disease widely considered a synonym for death is experienced as something to hide. The policy of equivocating about the nature of their disease with cancer patients reflects the conviction that dying people are best spared the news that they are dying, and that the good death is the sudden one, best of all if it happens while we're unconscious or asleep. Yet the modern denial of death does not explain the extent of the lying and the wish to be lied to; it does not touch the deepest dread. Someone who has had a coronary is at least as likely to die of another one within a few years as someone with cancer is likely to die soon from cancer. But no one thinks of concealing the truth from a cardiac patient: there is nothing shameful about a heart attack. Cancer patients are lied to, not just because the disease is (or is thought to be) a death sentence, but because it is felt to be obscene – in the original meaning of that word: ill-omened, abominable, repugnant to the senses. Cardiac disease implies a weakness, trouble, failure that is mechanical; there is no disgrace, nothing of the taboo that once surrounded peoples afflicted with TB and still surrounds those who have cancer. The metaphors attached to TB and to cancer imply living processes of a particularly resonant and horrid kind.

Chapter Two

Throughout most of their history, the metaphoric uses of TB and cancer crisscross and overlap. The *Oxford English Dictionary* records 'consumption' in use as a synonym for pulmonary tuberculosis as early as 1398.* (John of Trevisa: 'Whan the blode is made thynne, soo folowyth consumpcyon and wastyng.') But the premodern understanding of cancer also invokes the notion of consumption. The OED gives as the early figurative definition of cancer: 'Anything that frets, corrodes, corrupts, or consumes slowly and secretly.' (Thomas Paynell in 1528: 'A canker is a melancolye impostume eatynge partes of the bodye.') The earliest literal definition of cancer is a growth, lump, or protuberance, and the disease's name – from the Greek *karkínos* and the Latin

* Godefroy's *Dictionnaire de l'ancienne langue française* cites Bernard de Gordon's *Pratiqum* (1495): '*Tisis, c'est ung ulcere du polmon qui consume tout le corp.*'

cancer, both meaning crab – was inspired, according to Galen, by the resemblance of an external tumor's swollen veins to a crab's legs, not, as many people think, because a metastatic disease crawls or creeps like a crab. But etymology indicates that tuberculosis was also once considered a type of abnormal extrusion: the word tuberculosis – from the Latin *tüberculum*, the diminutive of *tüber*, bump, swelling – means a morbid swelling, protuberance, projection, or growth.* Rudolf Virchow, who founded the the science of cellular pathology in the 1850s, thought of the tubercle as a tumor.

Thus, from late antiquity until quite recently, tuberculosis was – typologically – cancer. And cancer was described, like TB, as a process in which the body was consumed. The modern conceptions of the two diseases could not be set until the advent of cellular pathology. Only with the microscope was it possible to grasp the distinctiveness of cancer, as a type of cellular activity, and to understand that the disease did not always take the form of an external or even palpable tumor. (Before the mid nineteenth century, nobody could have

---

* The same etymology is given in the standard French dictionaries. '*La tubercule*' was introduced in the sixteenth century by Ambroise Paré from the Latin *tüberculum*, meaning '*petite bosse*' (little lump). In Diderot's *Encyclopédie*, the entry on tuberculosis (1765) cites the definition given by the English physician Richard Morton in his *Phthisiologia* (1689): '*des petits tumeurs qui paraissent sur la surface du corps.*' In French, all tiny surface tumors were once called '*tubercules*'; the word became limited to what we identify as TB only after Koch's discovery of the tubercle bacillus.

identified leukemia as a form of cancer.) And it was not possible definitively to separate cancer from TB until after 1882, when tuberculosis was discovered to be a bacterial infection. Such advances in medical thinking enabled the leading metaphors of the two diseases to become truly distinct and, for the most part, contrasting. The modern fantasy about cancer could then begin to take shape – a fantasy which from the 1920s on would inherit most of the problems dramatized by the fantasies about TB, but with the two diseases and their symptoms conceived in quite different, almost opposing ways.

TB is understood as a disease of one organ, the lungs, while cancer is understood as a disease that can turn up in any organ and whose outreach is the whole body.

TB is understood as a disease of extreme contrasts: white pallor and red flush, hyperactivity alternating with languidness. The spasmodic course of the disease is illustrated by what is thought of as the prototypical TB symptom, coughing. The sufferer is wracked by coughs, then sinks back, recovers breath, breathes normally; then coughs again. Cancer is a disease of growth (sometimes visible; more characteristically, inside), of abnormal, ultimately lethal growth that is measured, incessant, steady. Although there may be periods in which tumor growth is arrested (remissions), cancer produces no contrasts like the oxymorons of behaviour – febrile activity, passionate resignation – thought to be typical of TB. The tubercular is pallid some of the time; the pallor of the cancer patient is unchanging.

TB makes the body transparent. The X-rays, which are the standard diagnostic tool, permit one, often for the first time, to see one's inside – to become transparent to oneself. While TB is understood to be, from early on, rich in visible symptoms (progressive emaciation, coughing, languidness, fever), and can be suddenly and dramatically revealed (the blood on the handkerchief), in cancer the main symptoms are thought to be, characteristically, invisible – until the last stage, when it is too late. The disease, often discovered by chance or through a routine medical checkup, can be far advanced without exhibiting any appreciable symptoms. One has an opaque body that must be taken to a specialist to find out if it contains cancer. What the patient cannot perceive, the specialist will determine by analyzing tissues taken from the body. TB patients may see their X-rays or even possess them: the patients at the sanatorium in *The Magic Mountain* carry theirs around in their breast pockets. Cancer patients don't look at their biopsies.

TB was – still is – thought to produce spells of euphoria, increased appetite, exacerbated sexual desire. Part of the regimen for patients in *The Magic Mountain* is a second breakfast, eaten with gusto. Cancer is thought to cripple vitality, make eating an ordeal, deaden desire. Having TB was imagined to be an aphrodisiac, and to confer extraordinary powers of seduction. Cancer is considered to be de-sexualizing. But it is characteristic of TB that many of its symptoms are deceptive – liveliness that comes from enervation, rosy cheeks that look like a sign of health but come from fever – and an upsurge of vitality may be a sign of approaching death. (Such gushes of energy will generally be self-destructive, and may be destructive of others: recall the Old West legend of Doc Holliday, the tubercular gunfighter released from moral restraints by the ravages of his disease.) Cancer has only true symptoms.

TB is disintegration, febrilization, dematerialization; it is a disease of liquids – the body turning to phlegm and mucus and sputum and, finally, blood – and of air, of the need for better air. Cancer is degeneration, the body tissues turning to something hard. Alice James, writing in her journal a year before she died from cancer in 1892, speaks of 'this unholy granite substance in my breast.' But this lump is alive, a fetus with its own will. Novalis, in an entry written around 1798 for his encyclopedia project, defines cancers, along with gangrene, as 'full-fledged *parasites* – they grow, are engendered, engender, have their structure, secrete, eat.' Cancer is a demonic pregnancy. St. Jerome must have been thinking of a cancer when he wrote: 'The one there with his swollen belly is pregnant with his own death' (*'Alius tumenti aqualiculo mortem parturit'*). Though the course of both diseases is emaciating, losing weight from TB is understood very differently from losing weight from cancer. In TB the person is 'consumed,' burned up. In cancer, the patient is 'invaded' by alien cells, which multiply, causing an atrophy or blockage of bodily functions. The cancer patient 'shrivels' (Alice James's word) or 'shrinks' (Wilhelm Reich's word).

TB is a disease of time; it speeds up life, highlights it,

spiritualizes it. In both English and French, consumption 'gallops.' Cancer has stages rather than gaits; it is (eventually) 'terminal.' Cancer works slowly, insidiously: the standard euphemism in obituaries is that someone has 'died after a long illness.' Every characterization of cancer describes it as slow, and so it was first used metaphorically. 'The word of hem crepith as a kankir,' Wyclif wrote in 1382 (translating a phrase in II Timothy 2:17); and among the earliest figurative uses of cancer are as a metaphor for 'idleness' and 'sloth.'* Metaphorically, cancer is not so much a disease of time as a disease or pathology of space. Its principal metaphors refer to topography (cancer 'spreads' or 'proliferates' or is 'diffused'; tumors are surgically 'excised'), and its most dreaded consequence, short of death, is the mutilation or amputation of part of the body.

TB is often imagined as a disease of poverty and deprivation — of thin garments, thin bodies, unheated rooms, poor hygiene, inadequate food. The poverty may not be as literal as Mimi's garret in *La Bohème*; the tubercular Marguerite Gautier in *La Dame aux camélias* lives in luxury, but inside she is a waif. In contrast, cancer is a disease of middle-class life, a disease associated with affluence, with excess. Rich countries have the

---

* As cited in the OED, which gives an early figurative use of 'canker': 'that pestilent and most infectious canker, idlenesse' — T. Palfreyman, 1564. And of 'cancer' (which replaced 'canker' around 1700): 'Sloth is a Cancer, eating up that Time Princes should cultivate for Things sublime' — Edmund Ken, 1711.

highest cancer rates, and the rising incidence of the disease is seen as resulting, in part, from a diet rich in fat and proteins and from the toxic effluvia of the industrial economy that creates affluence. The treatment of TB is identified with the stimulation of appetite, cancer treatment with nausea and the loss of appetite. The undernourished nourishing themselves – alas, to no avail. The overnourished, unable to eat.

The TB patient was thought to be helped, even cured, by a change in environment. There was a notion that TB was a wet disease, a disease of humid and dank cities. The inside of the body became damp ('moisture in the lungs' was a favored locution) and had to be dried out. Doctors advised travel to high, dry places – the mountains, the desert. But no change of surroundings is thought to help the cancer patient. The fight is all inside one's own body. It may be, is increasingly thought to be, something in the environment that has caused the cancer. But once cancer is present, it cannot be reversed or diminished by a move to a better (that is, less carcinogenic) environment.

TB is thought to be relatively painless. Cancer is thought to be, invariably excruciatingly painful. TB is thought to provide an easy death, while cancer is the spectacularly wretched one. For over a hundred years TB remained the preferred way of giving death a meaning – an edifying, refined disease. Nineteenth-century literature is stocked with descriptions of almost symptomless, unfrightened, beatific deaths from TB, particularly of young people, such as Little Eva in *Uncle Tom's Cabin* and Dombey's son Paul in *Dombey and Son* and Smike in *Nicholas Nickleby*, where Dickens described TB as the 'dread disease' which 'refines' death.

> if its grosser aspect ... in which the struggle between soul and body is so gradual, quiet, and solemn, and the result so sure, that day by day, and grain by grain, the mortal part wastes and withers away, so that the spirit grows light and sanguine with its lightening load ... *

Contrast these ennobling, placid TB deaths with the ignoble, agonizing cancer deaths of Eugene Gant's father in Thomas Wolfe's *Of Time and the River* and of the sister in Bergman's film *Cries and Whispers*. The dying tubercular is pictured as made more beautiful and more soulful; the person dying of cancer is portrayed as robbed of all capacities of self-transcendence, humiliated by fear and agony.

These are contrasts drawn from the popular mythology of both diseases. Of course, many tuberculars died in terrible pain, and some people die of cancer feeling little or no pain to the end; the poor and the rich

---

* Nearly a century later, in his edition of Katherine Mansfield's posthumously published *Journal*, John Middleton Murry uses similar language to describe Mansfield on the last day of her life. 'I have never seen, nor shall I ever see, any one so beautiful as she was on that day; it was as though the exquisite perfection which was always hers had taken possession of her completely. To use her own words, the last grain of "sediment," the last "traces of earthly degradation," were departed for ever. But she had lost her life to save it.'

both get TB and cancer; and not everyone who has TB coughs. But the mythology persists. It is not just because pulmonary tuberculosis is the most common form of TB that most people think of TB, in contrast to cancer, as a disease of one organ. It is because the myths about TB do not fit the brain, larynx, kidneys, long bones, and other sites where the tubercle bacillus can also settle, but do have a close fit with the traditional imagery (breath, life) associated with the lungs.

While TB takes on qualities assigned to the lungs, which are part of the upper, spiritualized body, cancer is notorious for attacking parts of the body (colon, bladder, rectum, breast, cervix, prostate, testicles) that are embarrassing to acknowledge. Having a tumor generally arouses some feelings of shame, but in the hierarchy of the body's organs, lung cancer is felt to be less shameful than rectal cancer. And one non-tumor form of cancer now turns up in commercial fiction in the role once monopolized by TB, as the romantic disease which cuts off a young life. (The heroine of Erich Segal's *Love Story* dies of leukemia – the 'white' or TB-like form of the disease, for which no mutilating surgery can be proposed – not of stomach or breast cancer.) A disease of the lungs is, metaphorically, a disease of the soul.* Cancer, as

* The Goncourt brothers, in their novel *Madame Gervaisais* (1869), called TB 'this illness of the lofty and noble parts of the human being,' contrasting it with 'the diseases of the crude, base organs of the body, which clog and soil the patient's mind . . .' In Mann's early story 'Tristan,' the young wife has tuberculosis of the trachea: '. . . the trachea, and not the lungs thank God! But it is a

a disease that can strike anywhere, is a disease of the body. Far from revealing anything spiritual, it reveals that the body is, all too woefully, just the body.

Such fantasies flourish because TB and cancer are thought to be much more than diseases that usually are (or were) fatal. They are identified with death iself. In *Nicholas Nickleby*, Dickens apostrophized TB as the

> disease in which death and life are so strangely blended, that death takes the glow and hue of life, and life the gaunt and grisly form of death; disease which medicine never cured, wealth never warded off, or poverty could boast exemption from . . .

And Kafka wrote to Max Brod in October 1917 that he had 'come to think that tuberculosis . . . is no special disease, or not a disease that deserves a special name, but only the germ of death itself, intensified . . .' Cancer inspires similar speculations. Georg Groddeck, whose remarkable views on cancer in *The Book of the It* (1923) anticipate those of Wilhelm Reich, wrote:

> Of all the theories put forward in connection with cancer, only one has in my opinion survived the passage of time, namely, that cancer leads through definite stages to death. I mean by that that what is not fatal is not cancer. From that

------

question whether, if it had been the lungs the new patient could have looked any more pure and ethereal, any remoter from the concerns of this world, than she did now as she leaned back pale and weary in her chaste white-enamelled arm-chair, beside her robust husband, and listened to the conversation.'

you may conclude that I hold out no hope of a new method of curing cancer ... [only] the many cases of so-called cancer ...

For all the progress in treating cancer, many people still subscribe to Groddeck's equation: cancer = death. But the metaphors surrounding TB and cancer reveal much about the idea of the morbid, and how it has evolved from the nineteenth century (when TB was the most common cause of death) to our time (when cancer is the most dreaded disease). The Romantics moralized death in a new way: with the TB death, which dissolved the gross body, etherealized the personality, expanded consciousness. It was equally possible, through fantasies about TB, to aestheticize death. Thoreau, who had TB, wrote in 1852: 'Death and disease are often beautiful, like ... the hectic glow of consumption.' Nobody conceives of cancer the way TB was thought of – as a decorative, often lyrical death. Cancer is a rare and still scandalous subject for poetry; and it seems unimaginable to aestheticize the disease.

Chapter Three

The most striking similarity between the myths of TB and cancer is that both are, or were, understood as diseases of passion. Fever in TB was a sign of an inward burning; the tubercular is someone 'consumed' by ardor, that ardor leading to the dissolution of the body. The use of metaphors drawn from TB to describe love – the image of a 'diseased' love, of a passion that 'consumes' – long antedates the Romantic movement.* Starting with the Romantics, the image was inverted, and TB was conceived as a variant of the disease of love. In a heart-breaking letter of November 1, 1820 from Naples, Keats, forever separated from Fanny Brawne, wrote, 'If I had any chance of recovery [from tuberculosis], this passion

* As in Act II, Scene 2 of Sir George Etherege's play *The Man of Mode* (1676): 'When love grows diseas'd, the best thing we can do is to put it to a violent death; I cannot endure the torture of a lingring and consumptive passion.'

would kill me.' As a character in *The Magic Mountain* explains: 'Symptoms of disease are nothing but a disguised manifestation of the power of love; and all disease is only love transformed.'

As once TB was thought to come from too much passion afflicting the reckless and sensual, today many people believe that cancer is a disease of insufficient passion, afflicting those who are sexually repressed, inhibited, unspontaneous, incapable of expressing anger. These seemingly opposite diagnoses are actually not so different versions of the same view (and deserve, in my opinion, the same amount of credence). For both psychological accounts of a disease stress the insufficiency or the balking of vital energies. As much as TB was celebrated as a disease of passion, it was also regarded as a disease of repression. The high-minded hero of Gide's *The Immoralist* contracts TB (paralleling what Gide perceived to be his own story) because he has repressed his true sexual nature; when Michel accepts Life, he recovers. With this scenario, today, Michel would have to get cancer.

As cancer is now imagined to be the wages of repression, so TB was once explained as the ravages of frustration. What is called a liberated sexual life is believed by some people today to stave off cancer, for virtually the same reason that sex was often prescribed to tuberculars as a therapy. In *The Wings of the Dove*, Milly Theale's doctor advises a love affair as a cure for her TB; and it is when she discovers that her duplicitous suitor, Merton Densher, is secretly engaged to her friend

Kate Croy that she dies. And in his letter of November 1820, Keats exclaimed: 'My dear Brown, I should have had her when I was in health, and I should have remained well.'

According to the mythology of TB, there is generally some passionate feeling which provokes, which expresses itself in, a bout of TB. But the passions must be thwarted, the hopes blighted. And the passion, although usually love, could be a political or moral passion. At the end of Turgenev's *On the Eve* (1860), Insarov, the young Bulgarian revolutionary-in-exile who is the hero of the novel, realizes that he can't return to Bulgaria. In a hotel in Venice, he sickens with longing and frustration, gets TB, and dies.

According to the mythology of cancer, it is generally a steady repression of feeling that causes the disease. In the earlier, more optimistic form of this fantasy, the repressed feelings were sexual; now in a notable shift, the repression of violent feeling is imagined to cause cancer. The thwarted passion that killed Insarov was idealism. The passion that people think will give them cancer if they don't discharge it is rage. There are no modern Insarovs. Instead, there are cancerphobes like Norman Mailer, who recently explained that had he not stabbed his wife (and acted out 'a murderous nest of feeling') he would have gotten cancer and 'been dead in a few years himself.' It is the same fantasy that was once attached to TB, but in rather a nastier version.

The source for much of the current fancy that associates cancer with the repression of passion is Wilhelm

Reich, who defined cancer as a 'disease following emotional resignation – a bio-energetic shrinking, a giving up of hope.' Reich illustrated his influential theory with Freud's cancer, which he thought began when Freud, naturally passionate and 'very unhappily married,' yielded to resignation:

> He lived a very calm, quiet, decent family life, but there is little doubt that he was very much dissatisfied genitally. Both his resignation and his cancer were evidence of that. Freud had to give up, as a person. He had to give up his personal pleasures, his personal delights, in his middle years ... if my view of cancer is correct, you just give up, you resign – and, then, you shrink.

Tolstoy's 'The Death of Ivan Ilyich' is often cited as a case history of the link between cancer and characterological resignation. But the same theory has been applied to TB by Groddeck, who defined TB as

> the pining to die away. The desire must die away, then, the desire for the in and out, the up and down of erotic love, which is symbolized in breathing. And with the desire the lungs die away ... the body dies away ...*

As do accounts of cancer today, the typical accounts of

---

* The passage continues: '... because desire increases during the illness, because the guilt of the ever-repeated symbolic dissipation of semen in the sputum is continually growing greater, ... because the It allows pulmonary disease to bring beauty to the eyes and cheek, alluring poisons!'

TB in the nineteenth century all feature resignation as the cause of the disease. They also show how, as the disease advances, one *becomes* resigned – Mimi and Camille die because of their renunciation of love, beatified by resignation. Robert Louis Stevenson's autobiographical essay 'Ordered South,' written in 1874, describes the stages whereby the tubercular is 'tenderly weaned from the passion of life,' and an ostentatious resignation is characteristic of the rapid decline of tuberculars as reported at length in fiction. In *Uncle Tom's Cabin*, Little Eva dies with preternatural serenity, announcing to her father a few weeks before the end: 'My strength fades away every day, and I know I must go.' All we learn of Milly Theale's death in *The Wings of the Dove* is that 'she turned her face to the wall.' TB was represented as the prototypical passive death. Often it was a kind of suicide. In Joyce's 'The Dead,' Michael Furey stands in the rain in Gretta Conroy's garden the night before she leaves for the convent school; she implores him to go home; 'he said he did not want to live' and a week later he dies.

TB sufferers may be represented as passionate but are, more characteristically, deficient in vitality, in life force. (As in the contemporary updating of this fantasy, the cancer-prone are those who are not sufficiently sensual or in touch with their anger.) This is how those two famously tough-minded observers, the Goncourt brothers, explain the TB of their friend Murger (the author of *Scènes de la vie de Bohème*): he is dying 'for want of vitality with which to withstand suffering.'

Michael Furey was 'very delicate,' as Gretta Conroy explains to her 'stout, tallish,' virile, suddenly jealous husband. TB is celebrated as the disease of born victims, of sensitive, passive people who are not quite life-loving enough to survive. (What is hinted at by the yearning but almost somnolent belles of Pre-Raphaelite art is made explicit in the emaciated, hollow-eyed, tubercular girls depicted by Edvard Munch.) And while the standard representation of a death from TB places the emphasis on the perfected sublimation of feeling, the recurrent figure of the tubercular courtesan indicates that TB was also thought to make the sufferer sexy.

Like all really successful metaphors, the metaphor of TB was rich enough to provide for two contradictory applications. It described the death of someone (like a child) thought to be too 'good' to be sexual: the assertion of an angelic psychology. It was also a way of describing sexual feelings – while lifting the responsibility for libertinism, which is blamed on a state of objective, physiological decadence or deliquescence. It was both a way of describing sensuality and promoting the claims of passion and a way of describing repression and advertising the claims of sublimation, the disease inducing both a 'numbness of spirit' (Robert Louis Stevenson's words) and a suffusion of higher feelings. Above all, it was a way of affirming the value of being more conscious, more complex, psychologically. Health becomes banal, even vulgar.

Chapter Four

It seems that having TB had already acquired the associations of being romantic by the mid eighteenth century. In Act I, Scene 1 of Oliver Goldsmith's satire on life in the provinces, *She Stoops to Conquer* (1773), Mr Hardcastle is mildly remonstrating with Mrs Hardcastle about how much she spoils her loutish son by a former marriage, Tony Lumpkin:

MRS H.: And I am to blame? The poor boy was always too sickly to do any good. A school would be his death. When he comes to be a little stronger, who knows what a year or two's Latin may do to him?

MR H.: Latin for him! A cat and fiddle. No, no, the alehouse and the stable are the only schools he'll ever go to.

MRS H.: Well, we must not snub the poor boy now, for I believe we shan't have him long among us. Any body that looks in his face may see he's consumptive.

MR H.: Ay, if growing too fat be one of the symptoms.

MRS H.: He coughs sometimes.

MR H.: Yes, when his liquor goes the wrong way.

MRS H.: I'm actually afraid of his lungs.

MR H.: And truly so am I; for he sometimes whoops like a speaking trumpet – [TONY *hallooing, behind the Scenes*] – O there he goes – A very consumptive figure, truly.

This exchange suggests that the fantasy about TB was already a received idea, for Mrs Hardcastle is nothing but an anthology of clichés of the smart London world to which she aspires, and which was the audience of Goldsmith's play.* Goldsmith presumes that the TB myth is already widely disseminated – TB being, as it were, the anti-gout. For snobs and parvenus and social climbers, TB was one index of being genteel, delicate, sensitive. With the new mobility (social and geographical) made possible in the eighteenth century, worth and station are not given; they must be asserted. They were asserted through new notions about clothes ('fashion') and new attitudes toward illness. Both clothes (the outer garment of the body) and illness (a kind of interior décor of the body) became tropes for new attitudes toward the self.

* Goldsmith, who was trained as a doctor and practiced medicine for a while, had other clichés about TB. In his essay 'On Education' (1759) Goldsmith wrote that a diet lightly salted, sugared, and seasoned 'corrects any consumptive habits, not unfrequently found amongst the children of city parents.' Consumption is viewed as a habit, a disposition (if not an affectation), a weakness that must be strengthened and to which city people are more disposed.

Shelley wrote on July 27, 1820 to Keats, commiserating as one TB sufferer to another, that he has learned 'that you continue to wear a consumptive appearance.' This was no mere turn of phrase. Consumption was understood as a manner of appearing, and that appearance became a staple of nineteenth-century manners. It became rude to eat heartily. It was glamorous to look sickly. 'Chopin was tubercular at a time when good health was not chic,' Camille Saint-Saëns wrote in 1913. 'It was fashionable to be pale and drained. Princess Belgiojoso strolled along the boulevards . . . pale as death in person.' Saint-Saëns was right to connect an artist, Chopin, with the most celebrated *femme fatale* of the period, who did a great deal to popularize the tubercular look. The TB-influenced idea of the body was a new model for aristocratic looks – at a moment when aristocracy stops being a matter of power, and starts being mainly a matter of image. ('One can never be too rich. One can never be too thin,' the Duchess of Windsor once said.) Indeed, the romanticizing of TB is the first widespread example of that distinctively modern activity, promoting the self as an image. The tubercular look had to be considered attractive once it came to be considered a mark of distinction, of breeding. 'I cough continually!' Marie Bashkirtsev wrote in the once widely read *Journal*, which was published, after her death at twenty-four, in 1887. 'But for a wonder, far from making me look ugly, this gives me an air of languor that is very becoming.' What was once the fashion of aristocratic *femmes fatales* and aspiring young artists became, eventually, the province of fashion as such. Twentieth-century women's fashions (with their cult of thinness) are the last stronghold of the metaphors associated with the romanticizing of TB in the late eighteenth and early nineteenth centuries.

Many of the literary and erotic attitudes known as 'romantic agony' derive from tuberculosis and its transformation through metaphor. Agony became romantic in a stylized account of the disease's preliminary symptoms (for example, debility is transformed into languor) and the actual agony was simply suppressed. Wan, hollow-chested young women and pallid, rachitic young men vied with each other as candidates for this mostly (at that time) incurable, disabling, really awful disease. 'When I was young,' wrote Théophile Gautier, 'I could not have accepted as a lyrical poet anyone weighing more than ninety-nine pounds.' (Note that Gautier says lyrical poet, apparently resigned to the fact that novelists had to be made of coarser and bulkier stuff.) Gradually, the tubercular look, which symbolized an appealing vulnerability, a superior sensitivity, became more and more the ideal look for women – while great men of the mid and late nineteenth century grew fat, founded industrial empires, wrote hundreds of novels, made wars, and plundered continents.

One might reasonably suppose that this romanticization of TB was a merely literary transfiguration of the disease, and that in the era of its great depredations TB was probably thought to be disgusting – as cancer is now. Surely everyone in the nineteenth century knew about, for example, the stench in the breath of the consumptive person. (Describing their visit to the dying Murger, the Goncourts note 'the odor of rotting flesh in his bedroom.') Yet all the evidence indicates that the cult of TB was not simply an invention of romantic poets and opera librettists but a widespread attitude, and that the person dying (young) of TB really was perceived as a romantic personality. One must suppose that the reality of this terrible disease was no match for important new ideas, particularly about individuality. It is with TB that the idea of individual illness was articulated, along with the idea that people are made more conscious as they confront their deaths, and in the images that collected around the disease one can see emerging a modern idea of individuality that has taken in the twentieth century a more aggressive, if no less narcissistic, form. Sickness was a way of making people 'interesting' – which is how 'romantic' was originally defined. (Schlegel, in his essay 'On the Study of Greek Poetry' [1795], offers 'the interesting' as the ideal of modern – that is, romantic – poetry.) 'The ideal of perfect health,' Novalis wrote in a fragment from the period 1799–1800, 'is only scientifically interesting'; what is really interesting is sickness, 'which belongs to individualizing.' This idea – of how interesting the sick are – was given its boldest and most ambivalent formulation by Nietzsche in *The Will to Power* and other writings, and though Nietzsche rarely mentioned a specific illness, those famous judgments about individual weakness and cultural exhaustion or decadence incorporate and extend many of the clichés about TB.

31

The romantic treatment of death asserts that people were made singular, made more interesting, by their illness. 'I look pale,' said Byron, looking into the mirror. 'I should like to die of a consumption.' 'Why?' asked a friend, who was visiting Byron in Athens in October 1810. 'Because the ladies would all say, "Look at that poor Byron, how interesting he looks in dying."' Perhaps the main gift to sensibility made by the Romantics is not the aesthetics of cruelty and the beauty of the morbid (as Mario Praz suggested in his famous book), or even the demand for unlimited personal liberty, but the nihilistic and sentimental idea of 'the interesting.'

Sadness made one 'interesting.' It was a mark of refinement, of sensibility, to be sad. That is, to be powerless. In Stendhal's *Armance*, the anxious mother is reassured by the doctor that Octave is not, after all, suffering from tuberculosis but only from that 'dissatisfied and critical melancholy characteristic of young people of his generation and position.' Sadness and tuberculosis became synonymous. The Swiss writer Henri Amiel, himself tubercular, wrote in 1852 in his *Journal intime*:

> Sky draped in gray, pleated by subtle shading, mists trailing on the distant mountains; nature despairing, leaves falling on all sides like the lost illusions of youth under the tears of incurable grief . . . The fir tree, alone in its vigour, green, stoical in the midst of this universal tuberculosis.

But it takes a sensitive person to feel such sadness; or by implication, to contract tuberculosis. The myth of TB constitutes the next-to-last episode in the long career of the ancient idea of melancholy – which was the artist's disease, according to the theory of the four humors. The melancholy character – or the tubercular – was a superior one: sensitive, creative, a being apart. Keats and Shelley may have suffered atrociously from the disease. But Shelley consoled Keats that 'this consumption is a disease particularly fond of people who write such good verses as you have done . . .' So well established was the cliché which connected TB and creativity that at the end of the century one critic suggested that it was the progressive disappearance of TB which accounted for the current decline of literature and the arts.

But the myth of TB provided more than an account of creativity. It supplied an important model of bohemian life, lived with or without the vocation of the artist. The TB sufferer was a dropout, a wanderer in endless search of the healthy place. Starting in the early nineteenth century, TB became a new reason for exile, for a life that was mainly traveling. (Neither travel nor isolation in a sanatorium was a form of treatment for TB before then.) There were special places thought to be good for tuberculars: in the early nineteenth century, Italy; then, islands in the Mediterranean, or the South Pacific; in the twentieth century, the mountains, the desert – all landscapes that had themselves been successively romanticized. Keats was advised by his doctors to move to Rome; Chopin tried the islands of the western Mediterranean; Robert Louis Stevenson chose a Pacific exile; D. H. Lawrence roamed over half the globe.* The Romantics invented invalidism as a pretext for leisure, and for dismissing bourgeois obligations in order to live only for one's art. It was a way of retiring from the world without having to take responsibility for the decision — the story of *The Magic Mountain*. After passing his exams and before taking up his job in a Hamburg ship-building firm, young Hans Castorp makes a three-week visit to his tubercular cousin in the sanatorium at Davos. Just before Hans 'goes down,' the doctor diagnoses a spot on his lungs. He stays on the mountain for the next seven years.

By validating so many possibly subversive longings and turning them into cultural pieties, the TB myth survived irrefutable human experience and accumulating

---

* 'By a curious irony,' Stevenson wrote, 'the places to which we are sent when health deserts us are often singularly beautiful . . . [and] I daresay the sick man is not very inconsolable when he receives sentence of banishment and is inclined to regard his ill-health as not the least fortunate accident of his life.' But the experience of such enforced banishment, as Stevenson went on to describe it, was something less agreeable. The tubercular cannot enjoy his good fortune: 'the world is disenchanted for him.'

Katherine Mansfield wrote: 'I seem to spend half of my life arriving at strange hotels . . . The strange door shuts upon the stranger, and then I slip down in the sheets. Waiting for the shadows to come out of the corners and spin their slow, slow web over the Ugliest Wallpaper of All . . . The man in the room next to mine has the same complaint as I. When I wake in the night I hear him turning. And then he coughs. And after a silence I cough. And he coughs again. This goes on for a long time. Until I feel we are like two roosters calling each other at false dawns. From far-away hidden farms.'

medical knowledge for nearly two hundred years. Although there was a certain reaction against the Romantic cult of the disease in the second half of the last century, TB retained most of its romantic attribute – as the sign of a superior nature, as a becoming frailty – through the end of the century and well into ours. It is still the sensitive young artist's disease in O'Neill's *Long Day's Journey into Night*. Kafka's letters are a compendium of speculations about the meaning of tuberculosis, as is *The Magic Mountain*, published in 1924, the year Kafka died. Much of the irony of *The Magic Mountain* turns on Hans Castorp, the stolid burgher, getting TB, the artist's disease – for Mann's novel is a late, self-conscious commentary on the myth of TB. But the novel still reflects the myth: the burgher *is* indeed spiritually refined by his disease. To die of TB was still mysterious and (often) edifying and remained so until practically nobody in Western Europe and North America died of it any more. Although the incidence of the disease began to decline precipitously after 1900 because of improved hygiene, the mortality rate among those who contracted it remained high; the power of the myth was dispelled only when proper treatment was finally developed, with the discovery of streptomycin in 1944 and the introduction of isoniazid in 1952.

If it is still difficult to imagine how the reality of such a dreadful disease could be transformed so preposterously, it may help to consider our own era's comparable act of distortion, under the pressure of the need to express romantic attitudes about the self. The object of distortion is not, of course, cancer – a disease which nobody has managed to glamorize (though it fulfills some of the functions as a metaphor that TB did in the nineteenth century). In the twentieth century, the repellent, harrowing disease that is made the index of a superior sensitivity, the vehicle of 'spiritual' feelings and 'critical' discontent, is insanity.

The fancies associated with tuberculosis and insanity have many parallels. With both illnesses, there is confinement. Sufferers are sent to a 'sanatorium' (the common word for a clinic for tuberculars and the most common euphemism for an insane asylum). Once put away, the patient enters a duplicate world with special rules. Like TB, insanity is a kind of exile. The metaphor of the psychic voyage is an extension of the romantic idea of travel that was associated with tuberculosis. To be cured, the patient had to be taken out of his or her daily routine. It is not an accident that the most common metaphor for an extreme psychological experience viewed positively – whether produced by drugs or by becoming psychotic – is a trip.

In the twentieth century the cluster of metaphors and attitudes formerly attached to TB split up and are parceled out to two diseases. Some features of TB go to insanity: the notion of the sufferer as a hectic, reckless creature of passionate extremes, someone too sensitive to bear the horrors of the vulgar, everyday world. Other features of TB go to cancer – the agonies that can't be romanticized. Not TB but insanity is the current vehicle of our secular myth of self-transcendence. The romantic view is that illness exacerbates consciousness. Once that illness was TB; now it is insanity that is thought to bring consciousness to a state of paroxysmic enlightenment. The romanticizing of madness reflects in the most vehement way the contemporary prestige of irrational or rude (spontaneous) behavior (acting-out), of that very passionateness whose repression was once imagined to cause TB, and is now thought to cause cancer.

Chapter Five

In 'Death in Venice,' passion brings about the collapse of all that has made Gustav von Aschenbach singular – his reason, his inhibitions, his fastidiousness. And disease further reduces him. At the end of the story, Aschenbach is just another cholera victim, his last degradation being to succumb to the disease afflicting so many in Venice at that moment. When in *The Magic Mountain* Hans Castorp is discovered to have tuberculosis, it is a promotion. His illness will make Hans become more singular, will make him more intelligent than he was before. In one fiction, disease (cholera) is the penalty for a secret love; in the other, disease (TB) is its expression. Cholera is the kind of fatality that, in retrospect, has simplified a complex self, reducing it to sick environment. The disease that individualizes, that sets a person in relief against the environment, is tuberculosis.

What once made TB seem so 'interesting' – or, as it was usually put, romantic – also made it a curse and a source of special dread. In contrast to the great epidemic diseases of the past (bubonic plague, typhus, cholera), which strike each person as a member of an afflicted community, TB was understood as a disease that isolates one from the community. However steep its incidence in a population, TB – like cancer today – always seemed to be a mysterious disease of individuals, a deadly arrow that could strike anyone, that singled out its victims one by one.

As after a cholera death, it used to be common practice to burn the clothes and other effects of someone who died of TB. 'Those brutal Italians have nearly finished their monstrous business,' Keats's companion Joseph Severn wrote from Rome on March 6, 1821, two weeks after Keats died in the little room on the Piazza di Spagna. 'They have burned all the furniture – and are now scraping the walls – making new windows – new doors – and even a new floor.' But TB was frightening, not only as a contagion, like cholera, but as a seemingly arbitrary, uncommunicable 'taint.' And people could believe that TB was inherited (think of the disease's recurrence in the families of Keats, the Brontës, Emerson, Thoreau, Trollope) and also believe that it revealed something singular about the person afflicted. In a similar way, the evidence that there are cancer-prone families and, possibly, a hereditary factor in cancer can be acknowledged without disturbing the belief that cancer is a disease that strikes each person, punitively, as an individual. No one asks, 'Why me?' who gets cholera or typhus. But 'Why me?' (meaning 'it's not fair') is the question of many who learn they have cancer.

However much TB was blamed on poverty and insalubrious surroundings, it was still thought that a certain inner disposition was needed in order to contract the disease. Doctors and laity believed in a TB character type – as now the belief in a cancer-prone character type, far from being confined to the back yard of folk superstition, passes for the most advanced medical thinking. In contrast to the modern bogey of the cancer-prone character – someone unemotional, inhibited, repressed – the TB-prone character that haunted imaginations in the nineteenth century was an amalgam of two different fantasies: someone both passionate and repressed.

That other notorious scourge among nineteenth-century diseases, syphilis, was at least not mysterious. Contracting syphilis was a predictable consequence, the consequence, usually, of having sex with a carrier of the disease. So, among all the guilt-embroidered fantasies about sexual pollution attached to syphilis, there was no place for a type of personality supposed to be especially susceptible to the disease (as was once imagined for TB and is now for cancer). The syphilitic personality type was someone who had the disease (Osvald in Ibsen's *Ghosts*, Adrian Leverkühn in *Doctor Faustus*), not someone who was likely to get it. In its role as scourge, syphilis implied a moral judgment (about off-limits sex, about prostitution) but not a psychological one. TB, once so mysterious – as cancer is now – suggested judgments of a deeper kind, both moral and psychological, about the ill.

*

The speculations of the ancient world made disease most often an instrument of divine wrath. Judgment was meted out either to a community (the plague in Book I of the *Iliad* that Apollo inflicts on the Achaeans in punishment for Agamemnon's abduction of Chryses' daughter; the plague in Oedipus that strikes Thebes because of the polluting presence of the royal sinner) or to a single person (the stinking wound in Philoctetes' foot). The diseases around which the modern fantasies have gathered — TB, cancer — are viewed as forms of self-judgment, of self-betrayal.

One's mind betrays one's body. 'My head and lungs have come to an agreement without my knowledge,' Kafka said about his TB in a letter to Max Brod in September 1917. Or one's body betrays one's feelings, as in Mann's late novel *The Black Swan*, whose aging heroine, youthfully in love with a young man, takes as the return of her menses what is actually a hemorrhage and the symptom of incurable cancer. The body's treachery is thought to have its own inner logic. Freud was 'very beautiful . . . when he spoke,' Wilhelm Reich reminisced. 'Then it hit him just here, in the mouth. And that is where my interest in cancer began.' That interest led Reich to propose his version of the link between a mortal disease and the character of those it humiliates.

In the pre-modern view of disease, the role of character was confined to one's behavior after its onset. Like any extreme situation, dreaded illnesses bring out both people's worst and best. The standard accounts of epidemics, however, are mainly of the devastating effect of disease upon character. The weaker the chronicler's pre-conception of disease as a punishment for wickedness, the more likely that the account will stress the moral corruption made manifest by the disease's spread. Even if the disease is not thought to be a judgment on the community, it becomes one – retroactively – as it sets in motion an inexorable collapse of morals and manners. Thucydides relates the ways in which the plague that broke out in Athens in 430 B.C. spawned disorder and lawlessness ('The pleasure of the moment took the place both of honor and expedience') and corrupted language itself. And the whole point of Boccaccio's description in the first pages of the *Decameron* of the great plague of 1348 is how badly the citizens of Florence behaved.

In contrast to this disdainful knowledge of how most loyalties and loves shatter in the panic produced by epidemic disease, the accounts of modern diseases – where the judgment tends to fall on the individual rather than the society – seem exaggeratedly unaware of how poorly many people take the news that they are dying. Fatal illness has always been viewed as a test of moral character, but in the nineteenth century there is a great reluctance to let anybody flunk the test. And the virtuous only become more so as they slide toward death. This is standard achievement for TB deaths in fiction, and goes with the inveterate spiritualizing of TB and the senti-mentalizing of its horrors. Tuberculosis provided a redemptive death for the fallen, like the young prostitute Fantine in *Les Misérables*, or a sacrificial death for the virtuous, like the heroine of Selma Lagerlöf's *The*

Phantom Chariot. Even the ultra-virtuous, when dying of this disease, boost themselves to new moral heights. *Uncle Tom's Cabin*: Little Eva during her last days urges her father to become a serious Christian and free his slaves. *The Wings of the Dove*: after learning that her suitor is a fortune hunter, Milly Theale wills her fortune to him and dies. *Dombey and Son*: 'From some hidden reason, very imperfectly understood by himself – if understood at all – [Paul] felt a gradually increasing impulse of affection, towards almost everything and everybody in the place.'

For those characters treated less sentimentally, the disease is viewed as the occasion finally to behave well. At the least, the calamity of disease can clear the way for insight into lifelong self-deceptions and failures of character. The lies that muffle Ivan Ilyich's drawn-out agony – his cancer being unmentionable to his wife and children – reveal to him the lie of his whole life; when dying, he is, for the first time, in a state of truth. The sixty-year-old civil servant in Kurosawa's film *Ikiru* (1952) quits his job after learning he has terminal stomach cancer and, taking up the cause of a slum neighborhood, fights the bureaucracy he had served. With one year to live, Watanabe wants to do something that is worthwhile, wants to redeem his mediocre life.

Chapter Six

Disease occurs in the *Iliad* and the *Odyssey* as supernatural punishment, as demonic possession, and as the result of natural causes. For the Greeks, disease could be gratuitous or it could be deserved (for a personal fault, a collective transgression, or a crime of one's ancestors). With the advent of Christianity, which imposed more moralized notions of disease, as of everything else, a closer fit between disease and 'victim' gradually evolved. The idea of disease as punishment yielded the idea that a disease could be a particularly appropriate and just punishment. Cresseid's leprosy in Henryson's *The Testament of Cresseid* and Madame de Merteuil's smallpox in *Les Liaisons dangereuses* show the true face of the beautiful liar – a most involuntary revelation.

In the nineteenth century, the notion that the disease fits the patient's character, as the punishment fits the sinner, was replaced by the notion that it expresses character. Disease can be challenged by the will. 'The will exhibits itself as organized body,' wrote Schopenhauer, but he denied that the will itself could be sick. Recovery from a disease depends on the will assuming 'dictatorial power in order to subsume the rebellious forces' of the body. One generation earlier, a great physician, Bichat, had used a similar image, calling health 'the silence of organs,' disease 'their revolt.' Disease is what speaks through the body, a language for dramatizing the mental: a form of self-expression. Groddeck described illness as 'a symbol, a representation of something going on within, a drama staged by the It . . .'*

According to the pre-modern ideal of a well-balanced character, expressiveness is supposed to be limited. Behavior is defined by its potentiality for excess. Thus, when Kant makes figurative use of cancer, it is a metaphor for excess feeling. 'Passions are cancers for pure practical reason and often incurable,' Kant wrote in *Anthropologie* (1798). 'The passions are . . . unfortunate moods that are pregnant with many evils,' he added, evoking the ancient metaphoric connections between cancer and a pregnancy. When Kant compares passions (that is, extreme feelings) to cancers, he is of course using the pre-modern sense of the disease and a

* Kafka, after his TB was diagnosed in September 1917, wrote in his diary: '. . . the infection in your lungs is only a symbol,' the symbol of an emotional 'wound whose inflammation is called F[elice] . . .' To Max Brod he wrote: 'the illness is speaking for me because I have asked it to do so'; and to Felice: 'Secretly I don't believe this illness to be tuberculosis, at least not primarily tuberculosis, but rather a sign of my general bankruptcy.'

pre-Romantic evaluation of passion. Soon, turbulent feeling was to be viewed much more positively. 'There is no one in the world less able to conceal his feelings than Emile,' said Rousseau – meaning it as a compliment.

As excess feelings become positive, they are no longer analogized – in order to denigrate them – to a terrible disease. Instead, disease is seen as the vehicle of excess feeling. TB is the disease that makes manifest intense desire; that discloses, in spite of the reluctance of the individual, what the individual does not want to reveal. The contrast is no longer between moderate passions and excessive ones but between hidden passions and those which are brought into the open. Illness reveals desires of which the patient probably was unaware. Diseases – and patients – become subjects for decipherment. And these hidden passions are now considered a source of illness. 'He who desires but acts not, breeds pestilence,' Blake wrote: one of his defiant Proverbs of Hell.

The early Romantic sought superiority by desiring, and by desiring to desire, more intensely than others do. The inability to realize these ideals of vitality and perfect spontaneity was thought to make someone an ideal candidate for TB. Contemporary romanticism starts from the inverse principle – that it is others who desire intensely, and that it is oneself (the narratives are typically in the first person) who has little or no desire at all. There are precursors of the modern romantic egos of unfeeling in nineteenth-century Russian novels (Pechorin in Lermontov's *A Hero of Our Time*, Stavrogin in *The Possessed*); but they are still heroes – restless, bitter, self-destructive, tormented by their inability to feel. (Even their glum, merely self-absorbed descendants, Roquentin in Sartre's *Nausea* and Meursault in Camus's *The Stranger*, seemed bewildered by their inability to feel.) The passive, affectless anti-hero who dominates contemporary American fiction is a creature of regular routines or unfeeling debauch; not self-destructive but prudent; not moody, dashing, cruel, just dissociated. The ideal candidate, according to contemporary mythology, for cancer.

Ceasing to consider disease as a punishment which fits the objective moral character, making it an expression of the inner self, might seem less moralistic. But this view turns out to be just as, or even more, moralistic and punitive. With the modern diseases (once TB, now cancer), the romantic idea that the disease expresses the character is invariably extended to assert that the character causes the disease – because it has not expressed itself. Passion moves inward, striking and blighting the deepest cellular recesses.

'The sick man himself creates his disease,' Groddeck wrote; 'he is the cause of the disease and we need seek none other.' 'Bacilli' heads Groddeck's list of mere 'external causes' – followed by 'chills, overeating, overdrinking, work, and anything else.' He insists that it is 'because it is not pleasant to look within ourselves' that doctors prefer to 'attack the outer causes with prophylaxis, disinfection, and so on,' rather than address the real, internal causes. In Karl Menninger's more recent formulation: 'Illness is in part what the world has done to a victim, but in larger part it is what the victim has done with his world, and with himself . . .' Such preposterous and dangerous views manage to put the onus of the disease on the patient and not only weaken the patient's ability to understand the range of plausible medical treatment but also, implicitly, direct the patient away from such treatment. Cure is thought to depend principally on the patient's already sorely tested or enfeebled capacity for self-love. A year before her death in 1923, Katherine Mansfield wrote in her *Journal*:

> A bad day . . . horrible pains and so on, and weakness. I could do nothing. The weakness was not only physical. I *must heal my Self* before I will be well . . . This must be done alone and at once. It is at the root of my not getting better. My mind is not *controlled*.

Mansfield not only thinks it was the 'Self' which made her sick but thinks that she has a chance of being cured of her hopelessly advanced lung disease if she could heal that 'Self.'*

Both the myth about TB and the current myth about cancer propose that one is responsible for one's disease.

* Mansfield, wrote John Middleton Murry, 'had come to the conviction that her bodily health depended upon her spiritual condition. Her mind was henceforth preoccupied with discovering some way to 'cure her soul'; and she eventually resolved, to my regret, to abandon her treatment and to live as though her grave physical illness were incidental, and even, so far as she could, as though it were nonexistent.'

But the cancer imagery is far more punishing. Given the romantic values in use for judging character and disease, some glamor attaches to having a disease thought to come from being full of passion. But there is mostly shame attached to a disease thought to stem from the repression of emotion – an opprobrium echoed in the views propagated by Groddeck and Reich, and the many writers influenced by them. The view of cancer as a disease of the failure of expressiveness condemns the cancer patient: expresses pity but also conveys contempt. Miss Gee, in Auden's poem from the 1930s, 'passed by the loving couples' and 'turned her head away.' Then:

> Miss Gee knelt down in the side-aisle,
>   She knelt down on her knees;
> 'Lead me not into temptation
>   But make me a good girl, please.'

> The days and nights went by her
>   Like waves round a Cornish wreck;
> She bicycled down to the doctor
>   With her clothes buttoned up to her neck.

> She bicycled down to the doctor,
>   And rang the surgery bell;
> 'O, doctor, I've pain inside me,
>   And I don't feel very well.'

> Doctor Thomas looked her over,
>   And then he looked some more;
> Walked over to his wash-basin,
>   Said, 'Why didn't you come before?'

Doctor Thomas sat over his dinner,
  Though his wife was waiting to ring,
Rolling his bread into pellets;
  Said, 'Cancer's a funny thing.

'Nobody knows what the cause is,
  Though some pretend they do;
It's like some hidden assassin
  Waiting to strike at you.

'Childless women get it,
  And men when they retire;
It's as if there had to be some outlet
  For their foiled creative fire.' . . .

The tubercular could be an outlaw or a misfit; the cancer personality is regarded more simply, and with condescension, as one of life's losers. Napoleon, Ulysses S. Grant, Robert A. Taft, and Hubert Humphrey have all had their cancer diagnosed as the reaction to political defeat and the curtailing of their ambitions. And the cancer deaths of those harder to describe as losers, like Freud and Wittgenstein, have been diagnosed as the gruesome penalty exacted for a lifetime of instinctual renunciation. (Few remember that Rimbaud died of cancer.) In contrast, the disease that claimed the likes of Keats, Poe, Chekhov, Simone Weil, Emily Brontë, and Jean Vigo was as much apotheosis as a verdict of failure.

Chapter Seven

Cancer is generally thought an inappropriate disease for a romantic character, in contrast to tuberculosis, perhaps because unromantic depression has supplanted the romantic notion of melancholy. 'A fitful strain of melancholy,' Poe wrote, 'will ever be found inseparable from the perfection of the beautiful.' Depression is melancholy minus its charms – the animation, the fits.

Supporting the theory about the emotional causes of cancer, there is a growing literature and body of research: and scarcely a week passes without a new article announcing to some general public or other the scientific link between cancer and painful feelings. Investigations are cited – most articles refer to the same ones – in which out of, say, several hundred cancer patients, two-thirds or three-fifths report being depressed or unsatisfied with their lives, and having suffered from the loss (through death or rejection or separation) of a parent, lover, spouse, or close friend. But it seems likely that of several hundred people who do *not* have cancer, most would also report depressing emotions and past traumas: this is called the human condition. And these case histories are recounted in a particularly forthcoming language of despair, of discontent about and obsessive preoccupation with the isolated self and its never altogether satisfactory 'relationships,' which bears the unmistakable stamp of our consumer culture. It is a language many Americans now use about themselves.*

Investigations carried out by a few doctors in the last

* A study by Dr. Caroline Bedell Thomas of the Johns Hopkins University School of Medicine was thus summarized in one recent newspaper article ('Can Your Personality Kill You?'): 'In brief, cancer victims are low-gear persons, seldom prey to outbursts of emotion. They have feelings of isolation from their parents dating back to childhood.' Drs Claus and Marjorie Bahnson at the Eastern Pennsylvania Psychiatric Institute have 'charted a personality pattern of denial of hostility, depression and of memory of emotional deprivation in childhood' and 'difficulty in maintaining close relationships.' Dr. O. Carl Simonton, a radiologist in Fort Worth, Texas, who gives patients both radiation and psychotherapy, describes the cancer personality as someone with 'a great tendency for self-pity and a markedly impaired ability to make and maintain meaningful relationships.' Lawrence LeShan, a New York psychologist and psychotherapist (*You Can Fight for Your Life: Emotional Factors in the Causation of Cancer* [1977]), claims that 'there is a general type of personality configuration among the majority of cancer patients' and a world-view that cancer patients share and 'which pre-dates the development of cancer.' He divides 'the basic emotional pattern of the cancer patient' into three parts: 'a childhood or adolescence marked by feelings of isolation,' the loss of the 'meaningful relationship' found in adulthood, and a subsequent 'conviction that life holds no more hope.' 'The cancer patient,' LeShan writes, 'almost invariably is contemptuous of himself, and of his abilities and possibilities.' Cancer patients are 'empty of feeling and devoid of self.'

century showed a high correlation between cancer and that era's complaints. In contrast to contemporary American cancer patients, who invariably report having feelings of isolation and loneliness since childhood, Victorian cancer patients described overcrowded lives, burdened with work and family obligations and bereavements. These patients don't express discontent with their lives as such or speculate about the quality of its satisfactions and the possibility of a 'meaningful relationship.' Physicians found the causes or predisposing factors of their patients' cancers in grief, in worry (noted as most acute among businessmen and the mothers of large families), in straitened economic circumstances and sudden reversals of fortune, and in overwork – or, if the patients were successful writers or politicians, in grief, rage, intellectual overexertion, the anxiety that accompanies ambition, and the stress of public life.*

---

* 'Always much trouble and hard work' is a notation that occurs in many of the brief case histories in Herbert Snow's *Clinical Notes on Cancer* (1883). Snow was a surgeon in the Cancer Hospital in London, and most of the patients he saw were poor. A typical observation: 'Of 140 cases of breast-cancer, 103 gave an account of previous mental trouble, hard work, or other debilitating agency. Of 187 uterine ditto, 91 showed a similar history.' Doctors who saw patients who led more comfortable lives made other observations. The physician who treated Alexandre Dumas for cancer, G. von Schmitt, published a book on cancer in 1871 in which he listed 'deep and sedentary study and pursuits, and feverish and anxious agitation of public life, the cares of ambition, frequent paroxysms of rage, violent grief' as 'the principal causes' of the disease. Quoted in Samuel J. Kowal, M.D., 'Emotions as a Cause of Cancer: 18th and 19th Century Contributions,' *Review of Psychoanalysis*, 42, 3 (July 1955).

Nineteenth-century cancer patients were thought to get the disease as the result of hyperactivity and hyper-intensity. They seemed to be full of emotions that had to be damped down. As a prophylaxis against cancer, one English doctor urged his patients 'to avoid over-taxing their strength, and to bear the ills of life with equanimity; above all things, not to "give way" to any grief.' Such stoic counsels have now been replaced by prescriptions for self-expression, from talking it out to the primal scream. In 1885, a Boston doctor advised 'those who have apparently benign tumors in the breast of the advantage of being cheerful.' Today, this would be regarded as encouraging the sort of emotional dissociation now thought to predispose people to cancer.

Popular accounts of the psychological aspects of cancer often cite old authorities, starting with Galen, who observed that 'melancholy women' are more likely to get breast cancer than 'sanguine women.' But the meanings have changed. Galen (second century A.D.) meant by melancholy a physiological condition with complex characterological symptoms; we mean a mere mood. 'Grief and anxiety,' said the English surgeon Sir Astley Cooper in 1845, are among 'the most frequent causes' of breast cancer. But the nineteenth-century observations undermine rather than support late-twentieth-century notions – evoking a manic or manic-depressive character type almost the op-posite of that forlorn, self-hating, emotionally inert creature, the contemporary cancer personality. As far as I know, no oncologist convinced of the efficacy of polychemotherapy and immunotherapy in treating patients has contributed to the fictions about a specific cancer personality. Needless to say, the hypothesis that distress can affect immunological responsiveness (and, in some circumstances, lower immunity to disease) is hardly the same as — or constitutes evidence for — the view that emotions cause diseases, much less for the belief that specific emotions can produce specific diseases.

Recent conjecture about the modern cancer character type finds its true antecedent and counterpart in the literature on TB, where the same theory, put in similar terms, had long been in circulation. In his *Morbidus Anglicus* (1672), Gideon Harvey declared 'Melancholy' and 'choler' to be 'the sole cause' of TB (for which he used the metaphoric term 'corrosion'). In 1881, a year before Robert Koch published his paper announcing the discovery of the tubercle bacillus and demonstrating that it was the primary cause of the disease, a standard medical textbook gave as the causes of tuberculosis: hereditary disposition, unfavorable climate, sedentary indoor life, defective ventilation, deficiency of light, and 'depressing emotions.'[*] Though the entry had to be changed for the next edition, it took a long time for these notions to lose credibility. 'I'm mentally ill, the disease of the lungs is nothing but an overflowing of my mental disease,' Kafka wrote to Milena in 1920. Applied to TB, the theory that

---

[*] August Flint and William H. Welch, *The Principles and Practice of Medicine* (fifth edition, 1881), cited in René and Jean Dubos, *The White Plague* (1952).

emotions cause diseases survived well into this century – until, finally, it was discovered how to cure the disease. The theory's fashionable current application – which relates cancer to emotional withdrawal and lack of self-confidence and confidence in the future – is likely to prove more tenable than its application to tuberculosis.

In the plague-ridden England of the late sixteenth and seventeenth centuries, according to the historian Keith Thomas, it was widely believed that 'the happy man would not get plague.' The fantasy that a happy state of mind would fend off disease probably flourished for all infectious diseases, before the nature of infection was understood. Theories that diseases are caused by mental states and can be cured by will power are always an index of how much is not understood about the physical terrain of a disease.

Moreover, there is a peculiarly modern predilection for psychological explanations of disease, as of everything else. Psychologizing seems to provide control over the experiences and events (like grave illnesses) over which people have in fact little or no control. Psychological understanding undermines the 'reality' of a disease. That reality has to be explained. (It really means; or is a symbol of; or must be interpreted so.) For those who live neither with religious consolations about death nor with a sense of death (or of anything else) as natural, death is the obscene mystery, the ultimate affront, the thing that cannot be controlled. It can only be denied. A large part of the popularity and persuasiveness of chology comes from its being a sublimated spiritualism: a secular, ostensibly scientific way of affirming the primacy of 'spirit' over matter. That ineluctably material reality, disease, can be given a psychological explanation. Death itself can be considered, ultimately, a psychological phenomenon. Groddeck declared in *The Book of the It* (he was speaking of TB): 'He alone will die who wishes to die, to whom life is intolerable.' The promise of a temporary triumph over death is implicit in much of the psychological thinking that starts from Freud and Jung.

At the least there is the promise of a triumph over illness. A 'physical' illness becomes in a way less real – but, in compensation, more interesting – so far as it can be considered a 'mental' one. Speculation throughout the modern period has tended steadily to enlarge the category of mental illness. Indeed, part of the denial of death in this culture is a vast expansion of the category of illness as such.

Illness expands by means of two hypotheses. The first is that every form of social deviation can be considered an illness. Thus, if criminal behavior can be considered an illness, then criminals are not to be condemned or punished but to be understood (as a doctor understands), treated, cured.* The second is that every illness can be

---

* An early statement of this view, now so much on the defensive, is in Samuel Butler's *Erewhon* (1872). Butler's way of suggesting that criminality was a disease, like TB, that was either hereditary or the result of an unwholesome environment was to point out the absurdity of condemning the sick. In Erewhon, those who murdered or stole are sympathetically treated as ill persons, while tuberculosis is punished as a crime.

considered psychologically. Illness is interpreted as, basically, a psychological event, and people are encouraged to believe that they get sick because they (unconsciously) want to, and that they can cure themselves by the mobilization of will; that they can choose not to die of the disease. These two hypotheses are complementary. As the first seems to relieve guilt, the second reinstates it. Psychological theories of illness are a powerful means of placing the blame on the ill. Patients who are instructed that they have, unwittingly, caused their disease are also being made to feel that they have deserved it.

Chapter Eight

Punitive notions of disease have a long history, and such notions are particularly active with cancer. There is the 'fight' or 'crusade' against cancer; cancer is the 'killer' disease; people who have cancer are 'cancer victims.' Ostensibly, the illness is the culprit. But it is also the cancer patient who is made culpable. Widely believed psychological theories of disease assign to the luckless ill the ultimate responsibility both for falling ill and for getting well. And conventions of treating cancer as no mere disease but a demonic enemy make cancer not just a lethal disease but a shameful one.

Leprosy in its heyday aroused a similarly disproportionate sense of horror. In the Middle Ages, the leper was a social text in which corruption was made visible; an exemplum, an emblem of decay. Nothing is more punitive than to give a disease a meaning – that meaning being invariably a moralistic one. Any important disease whose causality is murky, and for which treatment is

59

ineffectual, tends to be awash in significance. First, the subjects of deepest dread (corruption, decay, pollution, anomie, weakness) are identified with the disease. The disease itself becomes a metaphor. Then, in the name of the disease (that is, using it as a metaphor), that horror is imposed on other things. The disease becomes adjectival. Something is said to be disease-like, meaning that it is disgusting or ugly. In French, a mouldering stone façade is still *lépreuse*.

Epidemic diseases were a common figure for social disorder. From pestilence (bubonic plague) came 'pestilent,' whose figurative meaning, according to the *Oxford English Dictionary*, is 'injurious to religion, morals, or public peace – 1513'; and 'pestilential,' meaning 'morally baneful or pernicious – 1531.' Feelings about evil are projected onto a disease. And the disease (so enriched with meanings) is projected onto the world.

In the past, such grandiloquent fantasies were regularly attached to the epidemic diseases, diseases that were a collective calamity. In the last two centuries, the diseases most often used as metaphors for evil were syphilis, tuberculosis, and cancer – all diseases imagined to be, pre-eminently, the diseases of individuals.

Syphilis was thought to be not only a horrible disease but a demeaning, vulgar one. Anti-democrats used it to evoke the desecrations of an egalitarian age. Baudelaire, in a note for his never completed book on Belgium, wrote:

> We all have the republican spirit in our veins, like syphilis
> in our bones – we are democraticized and venerealized.

In the sense of an infection that corrupts morally and debilitates physically, syphilis was to become a standard trope in late-nineteenth- and early-twentieth-century anti-Semitic polemics. In 1933 Wilhelm Reich argued that 'the irrational fear of syphilis was one of the major sources of National Socialism's political views and its anti-Semitism.' But although he perceived sexual and political phobias being projected onto a disease in the grisly harping on syphilis in *Mein Kampf*, it never occurred to Reich how much was being projected in his own persistent use of cancer as a metaphor for the ills of the modern era. Indeed, cancer can be stretched much further than syphilis can as a metaphor.

Syphilis was limited as a metaphor because the disease itself was not regarded as mysterious; only awful. A tainted heredity (Ibsen's *Ghosts*), the perils of sex (Charles-Louis Philippe's *Bubu de Montparnasse*, Mann's *Doctor Faustus*) – there was horror aplenty in syphilis. But no mystery. Its causality was clear, and understood to be singular. Syphilis was the grimmest of gifts, 'transmitted' or 'carried' by a sometimes ignorant sender to the unsuspecting receiver. In contrast, TB was regarded as a mysterious affliction, and a disease with myriad causes – just as today, while everyone acknowledges cancer to be an unsolved riddle, it is also generally agreed that cancer is multi-determined. A variety of factors – such as cancer-causing substances ('carcinogens') in the environment, genetic makeup, lowering of immuno-defenses (by previous illness or emotional trauma), characterological predisposition – are held responsible for the disease. And many researchers assert that cancer is not one but more than a hundred clinically distinct diseases, that each cancer has to be studied separately, and that what will eventually be developed is an array of cures, one for each of the different cancers.

The resemblance of current ideas about cancer's myriad causes to long-held but now discredited views about TB suggests the possibility that cancer may be one disease after all and that it may turn out, as TB did, to have a principal causal agent and be controllable by one program of treatment. Indeed, as Lewis Thomas has observed, all the diseases for which the issue of causation has been settled, and which can be prevented and cured, have turned out to have a simple physical cause – like the pneumococcus for pneumonia, the tubercle bacillus for tuberculosis, a single vitamin deficiency for pellagra – and it is far from unlikely that something comparable will eventually be isolated for cancer. The notion that a disease can be explained only by a variety of causes is precisely characteristic of thinking about diseases whose causation is *not* understood. And it is diseases thought to be multi-determined (that is, mysterious) that have the widest possibilities as metaphors for what is felt to be socially or morally wrong.

TB and cancer have been used to express not only (like syphilis) crude fantasies about contamination but also fairly complex feelings about strength and weakness, and about energy. For more than a century and a half, tuberculosis provided a metaphoric equivalent for delicacy, sensitivity, sadness, powerlessness; while whatever seemed ruthless, implacable, predatory, could be analogized to cancer. (Thus, Baudelaire in 1852, in his essay, '*L'Ecole païenne*,' observed: 'A frenzied passion for art is a canker that devours the rest . . .') TB was an ambivalent metaphor, both a scourge and an emblem of refinement. Cancer was never viewed other than as a scourge; it was, metaphorically, the barbarian within.

While syphilis was thought to be passively incurred, an entirely involuntary disaster, TB was once, and cancer is now, thought to be a pathology of energy, a disease of the will. Concern about energy and feeling, fears about the havoc they wreak, have been attached to both diseases. Getting TB was thought to signify a defective vitality, or vitality misspent. 'There was a great want of vital power . . . and great constitutional weakness' – so Dickens described little Paul in *Dombey and Son*. The Victorian idea of TB as a disease of low energy (and heightened sensitivity) has its exact complement in the Reichian idea of cancer as a disease of unexpected energy (and anesthetized feelings). In an era in which there seemed to be no inhibitions on being productive, people were anxious about not having enough energy. In our own era of destructive overproduction by the economy and of increasing bureaucratic restraints on the individual, there is both a fear of having too much energy and an anxiety about energy not being allowed to be expressed.

Like Freud's scarcity-economics theory of 'instincts,' the fantasies about TB which arose in the last century (and lasted well into ours) echo the attitudes of early capitalist accumulation. One has a limited amount of energy, which must be properly spent. (Having an orgasm, in nineteenth-century English slang, was not 'coming' but 'spending.') Energy, like savings, can be depleted, can run out or be used up, through reckless expenditure. The body will start 'consuming' itself, the patient will 'waste away.'

The language used to describe cancer evokes a different economic catastrophe: that of unregulated, abnormal, incoherent growth. The tumor has energy, not the patient; 'it' is out of control. Cancer cells, according to the textbook account, are cells that have shed the mechanism which 'restrains' growth. (The growth of normal cells is 'self-limiting,' due to a mechanism called 'contact inhibition.') Cells without inhibitions, cancer cells will continue to grow and extend over each other in a 'chaotic' fashion, destroying the body's normal cells, architecture, and functions.

Early capitalism assumes the necessity of regulated spending, saving, accounting, discipline – an economy that depends on the rational limitation of desire. TB is described in images that sum up the negative behavior of nineteenth-century *homo economicus*: consumption; wasting; squandering of vitality. Advanced capitalism requires expansion, speculation, the creation of new needs (the problem of satisfaction and dissatisfaction); buying on credit; mobility – an economy that depends on the irrational indulgence of desire. Cancer is described in images that sum up the negative behavior of twentieth-century *homo economicus*: abnormal growth; repression of energy, that is, refusal to consume or spend.

TB was understood, like insanity, to be a kind of onesidedness: a failure of will or an overintensity. However much the disease was dreaded, TB always had pathos. Like the mental patient today, the tubercular was considered to be someone quintessentially vulnerable, and full of self-destructive whims. Nineteenth- and early-twentieth-century physicians addressed themselves to coaxing their tubercular patients back to health. Their prescription was the same as the enlightened one for mental patients today: cheerful surroundings, isolation from stress and family, healthy diet, exercise, rest.

The understanding of cancer supports quite different, avowedly brutal notions of treatment. (A common cancer hospital witticism, heard as often from doctors as from patients: 'The treatment is worse than the disease.') There can be no question of pampering the patient. With the patient's body considered to be under attack ('invasion'), the only treatment is counter-attack.

The controlling metaphors in descriptions of cancer are, in fact, drawn not from economics but from the language of warfare: every physician and every attentive patient is familiar with, if perhaps inured to, this military terminology. Thus, cancer cells do not simply multiply; they are 'invasive.' ('Malignant tumors invade even when they grow very slowly,' as one textbook puts it.)

Cancer cells 'colonize' from the original tumor to far sites in the body, first setting up tiny outposts ('micro-metastases') whose presence is assumed, though they cannot be detected. Rarely are the body's 'defenses' vigorous enough to obliterate a tumor that has established its own blood supply and consists of billions of destructive cells. However 'radical' the surgical intervention, however many 'scans' are taken of the body landscape, most remissions are temporary; the prospects are that 'tumor invasion' will continue, or that rogue cells will eventually regroup and mount a new assault on the organism.

Treatment also has a military flavor. Radiotherapy uses the metaphors of aerial warfare; patients are 'bombarded' with toxic rays. And chemotherapy is chemical warfare, using poisons.* Treatment aims to 'kill' cancer cells (without, it is hoped, killing the patient). Unpleasant

---

* Drugs of the nitrogen mustard type (so-called alkylating agents) – like cyclophosphamide (Cytoxan) – were the first generation of cancer drugs. Their use with leukemia (which is characterized by an excessive production of immature white cells), then with other forms of cancer – was suggested by an inadvertent experiment with chemical warfare toward the end of World War II, when an American ship, loaded with nitrogen mustard gas, was blown up in the Naples harbor, and many of the sailors died of their lethally low white-cell and platelet counts (that is, of bone-marrow poisoning) rather than of burns or sea-water inhalation.

Chemotherapy and weaponry seem to go together, if only as a fancy. The first modern chemotherapy success was with syphilis: in 1910, Paul Ehrlich introduced an arsenic derivative, arsphenamine (Salvarsan), which was called 'the magic bullet.'

side effects to treatment are advertised, indeed over-advertised. ('The agony of chemotherapy' is a standard phrase.) It is impossible to avoid damaging or destroying healthy cells (indeed, some methods used to treat cancer can cause cancer), but it is thought that nearly any damage to the body is justified if it saves the patient's life. Often, of course, it doesn't work. (As in: 'We had to destroy Ben Suc in order to save it.') There is everything but the body count.

The military metaphor in medicine first came into wide use in the 1880s, with the identification of bacteria as agents of disease. Bacteria were said to 'invade' or 'infiltrate.' But talk of siege and war to describe disease now has, with cancer, a striking literalness and authority. Not only is the clinical course of the disease and its medical treatment thus described, but the disease itself is conceived as the enemy on which society wages war. More recently, the fight against cancer has sounded like a colonial war — with similarly vast appropriations of government money — and in a decade when colonial wars haven't gone too well, this militarized rhetoric seems to be backfiring. Pessimism among doctors about the efficacy of treatment is growing, in spite of the strong advances in chemotherapy and immunotherapy made since 1970. Reporters covering 'the war on cancer' frequently caution the public to distinguish between official fictions and harsh facts; a few years ago, one science writer found American Cancer Society proclamations that cancer is curable and progress has been made 'reminiscent of Vietnam optimism prior to the deluge.'

Still, it is one thing to be skeptical about the rhetoric that surrounds cancer, another to give support to many uninformed doctors who insist that no significant progress in treatment has been made, and that cancer is not really curable. The bromides of the American cancer establishment, tirelessly hailing the imminent victory over cancer; the professional pessimism of a large number of cancer specialists, talking like battle-weary officers mired down in an interminable colonial war – these are twin distortions in this military rhetoric about cancer.

Other distortions follow with the extension of cancer images in more grandiose schemes of warfare. As TB was represented as the spiritualizing of consciousness, cancer is understood as the overwhelming or obliterating of consciousness (by a mindless It). In TB, you are eating yourself up, being refined, getting down to the core, the real you. In cancer, non-intelligent ('primitive,' 'embryonic,' 'atavistic') cells are multiplying, and you are being replaced by the nonyou. Immunologists class the body's cancer cells as 'nonself.'

It is worth noting that Reich, who did more than anyone else to disseminate the psychological theory of cancer, also found something equivalent to cancer in the biosphere.

> There is a deadly orgone energy. It is in the atmosphere. You can demonstrate it on devices such as the Geiger counter. It's a swampy quality ... Stagnant, deadly water which doesn't flow, doesn't metabolize. Cancer, too, is due to the stagnation of the flow of the life energy of the organism.

Reich's language has its own inimitable coherence. And more and more – as its metaphoric uses gain in credibility – cancer is felt to be what he thought it was, a cosmic disease, the emblem of all the destructive, alien powers to which the organism is host.

As TB was the disease of the sick self, cancer is the disease of the Other. Cancer proceeds by a science-fiction scenario: an invasion of 'alien' or 'mutant' cells, stronger than normal cells (*Invasion of the Body Snatchers, The Incredible Shrinking Man, The Blob, The Thing*). One standard science-fiction plot is mutation, either mutants arriving from outer space or accidental mutations among humans. Cancer could be described as a triumphant mutation, and mutation is now mainly an image for cancer. As a theory of the psychological genesis of cancer, the Reichian imagery of energy checked, not allowed to move outward, then turned back on itself, driving cells berserk, is already the stuff of science fiction. And Reich's image of death in the air – of deadly energy that registers on a Geiger counter – suggests how much the science-fiction images about cancer (a disease that comes from deadly rays, and is treated by deadly rays) echo the collective nightmare. The original fear about exposure to atomic radiation was genetic deformities in the next generation; that was replaced by another fear, as statistics started to show much higher cancer rates among Hiroshima and Nagasaki survivors and their descendants.

Cancer is a metaphor for what is most ferociously energetic; and these energies constitute the ultimate insult to natural order. In a science-fiction tale by Tommaso

Landolfi, the spaceship is called 'Cancerqueen.' (It is hardly within the range of the tuberculosis metaphor that a writer could have imagined an intrepid vessel named 'Consumptionqueen.') When not being explained away as something psychological, buried in the recesses of the self, cancer is being magnified and projected into a metaphor for the biggest enemy, the furthest goal. Thus, Nixon's bid to match Kennedy's promise to put Americans on the moon was, appropriately enough, the promise to 'conquer' cancer. Both were science-fiction ventures. The equivalent of the legislation establishing the space program was the National Cancer Act of 1971, which did not envisage the near-to-hand decisions that could bring under control the industrial economy that pollutes – only the great destination: the cure.

TB was a disease in the service of a romantic view of the world. Cancer is now in the service of a simplistic view of the world that can turn paranoid. The disease is often experienced as a form of demonic possession – tumors are 'malignant' or 'benign,' like forces – and many terrified cancer patients are disposed to seek out faith healers, to be exorcised. The main organized support for dangerous nostrums like Laetrile comes from far-right groups to whose politics of paranoia the fantasy of a miracle cure for cancer makes a serviceable addition, along with a belief in UFOs. (The John Birch Society distributes a forty-five-minute film called *World Without Cancer*.) For the more sophisticated, cancer signifies the rebellion of the injured ecosphere: Nature taking revenge on a wicked technocratic world. False hopes and simplified terrors are raised by crude statistics brandished for the general public, such as that 90 percent of all cancers are 'environmentally caused,' or that imprudent diet and tobacco smoking alone account for 75 percent of all cancer deaths. To the accompaniment of this numbers game (it is difficult to see how any statistics about 'all cancers' or 'all cancer deaths' could be defended), cigarettes, hair dyes, bacon, saccharine, hormone-fed poultry, pesticides, low-sulphur coal – a lengthening roll call of products we take for granted have been found to cause cancer. X-rays give cancer (the treatment meant to cure kills); so do emanations from the television set and the microwave oven and the fluorescent clock face. As with syphilis, an innocent or trivial act – or exposure – in the present can have dire consequences far in the future. It is also known that cancer rates are high for workers in a large number of industrial occupations. Though the exact processes of causation lying behind the statistics remain unknown, it seems clear that many cancers are preventable. But cancer is not just a disease ushered in by the Industrial Revolution (there was cancer in Arcadia) and certainly more than the sin of capitalism (within their more limited industrial capacities, the Russians pollute worse than we do). The widespread current view of cancer as a disease of industrial civilization is as unsound scientifically as the right-wing fantasy of a 'world without cancer' (like a world without subversives). Both rest on the mistaken feeling that cancer is a distinctively 'modern' disease.

The medieval experience of the plague was firmly

tied to notions of moral pollution, and people invariably looked for a scapegoat external to the stricken community. (Massacres of Jews in unprecedented numbers took place everywhere in plague-stricken Europe of 1347–8, then stopped as soon as the plague receded.) With the modern diseases, the scapegoat is not so easily separated from the patient. But much as these diseases individualize, they also pick up some of the metaphors of epidemic diseases. (Diseases understood to be simply epidemic have become less useful as metaphors, as evidenced by the near-total historical amnesia about the influenza pandemic of 1918–19, in which more people died than in the four years of World War I.) Presently, it is as much a cliché to say that cancer is 'environmentally' caused as it was – and still is – to say that it is caused by mismanaged emotions. TB was associated with pollution (Florence Nightingale thought it was 'induced by the foul air of houses'), and now cancer is thought of as a disease of the contamination of the whole world. TB was 'the white plague.' With awareness of environmental pollution, people have started saying that there is an 'epidemic' or 'plague' of cancer.

Chapter Nine

Illnesses have always been used as metaphors to enliven charges that a society was corrupt or unjust. Traditional disease metaphors are principally a way of being vehement; they are, compared with the modern metaphors, relatively contentless. Shakespeare does many variations on a standard form of the metaphor, an infection in the 'body politic' – making no distinction between a contagion, an infection, a sore, an abscess, an ulcer, and what we would call a tumor. For purposes of invective, diseases are of only two types: the painful but curable, and the possibly fatal. Particular diseases figure as examples of diseases in general; no disease has its own distinctive logic. Disease imagery is used to express concern for social order, and health is something everyone is presumed to know about. Such metaphors do not project the modern idea of a specific master illness, in which what is at issue is health itself.

Master illnesses like TB and cancer are more

specifically polemical. They are used to propose new, critical standards of individual health, and to express a sense of dissatisfaction with society as such. Unlike the Elizabethan metaphors – which complain of some general aberration of public calamity that is, in consequence, dislocating to individuals – the modern metaphors suggest a profound disequilibrium between individual and society, with a society conceived as the individual's adversary. Disease metaphors are used to judge society not as out of balance but as repressive. They turn up regularly in Romantic rhetoric which opposes heart to head, spontaneity to reason, nature to artifice, country to city.

When travel to a better climate was invented as a treatment for TB in the early nineteenth century, the most contradictory destinations were proposed. The south, mountains, deserts, islands – their very diversity suggests what they have in common: the rejection of the city. In *La Traviata*, as soon as Alfredo wins Violetta's love, he moves her from unhealthy wicked Paris to the wholesome countryside: instant health follows. And Violetta's giving up on happiness is tantamount to leaving the country and returning to the city – where her doom is sealed, her TB returns, and she dies.

The metaphor of cancer expands the theme of the rejection of the city. Before it was understood as, literally, a cancer-causing (carcinogenic) environment, the city was seen as itself a cancer – a place of abnormal, unnatural growth. In *The Living City* (1958), Frank Lloyd Wright compared the city of earlier times, a healthy organism ('The city then was not malignant'), with the modern city. 'To look at the cross-section of any plan of a big city is to look at the section of a fibrous tumor.'*

Throughout the nineteenth century, disease metaphors become more virulent, preposterous, demagogic. And there is an increasing tendency to call any situation one disapproves of a disease. Disease, which could be considered as much a part of nature as is health, became the synonym of whatever was 'unnatural.' In *Les Misérables*, Hugo wrote:

> Monasticism, such as it existed in Spain and as it exists in Tibet, is for civilization a sort of tuberculosis. It cuts off life. Quite simply, it depopulates. Confinement, castration. It was a scourge in Europe.

Bichat in 1800 defined life as 'the ensemble of functions which resists death.' That contrast between life and death was to be transferred to a contrast between life and disease. Disease (now equated with death) is what opposes life.

---

* The sociologist Herbert Gans has called my attention to the importance of tuberculosis and the alleged or real threat of it in the slum-clearing and 'model tenement' movements of the late nineteenth and early twentieth centuries, the feeling being that slum housing 'bred' TB. The shift from TB to cancer in planning and housing rhetoric had taken place by the 1950s. 'Blight' (a virtual synonym for slum) is seen as a cancer that spreads insidiously, and the use of the term 'invasion' to describe when the non-white and poor move into a middle-class neighborhood is as much a metaphor borrowed from cancer as from the military: the two discourses overlap.

In 1916, in 'Socialism and Culture,' Gramsci denounced

> the habit of thinking that culture is encyclopedic knowledge ... This form of culture serves to create that pale and broken-winded intellectualism ... which has produced a whole crowd of boasters and day-dreamers more harmful to a healthy social life than tuberculosis or syphilis microbes are to the body's beauty and health ...

In 1919, Mandelstam paid the following tribute to Pasternak:

> To read Pasternak's verse is to clear one's throat, to fortify one's breathing, to fill one's lungs; such poetry must be healthy, a cure for tuberculosis. No poetry is healthier at the present moment. It is like drinking *koumiss* after canned American milk.

And Marinetti, denouncing Communism in 1920:

> Communism is the exasperation of the bureaucratic cancer that has always wasted humanity. A German cancer, a product of the characteristic German preparationism. Every pedantic preparation is anti-human ...

It is for the same iniquity that the protofascist Italian writer attacks Communism and the future founder of the Italian Communist Party attacks a certain bourgeois idea of culture ('truly harmful, especially to the proletariat,' Gramsci says) – for being artificial, pedantic, rigid, lifeless. Both TB and cancer have been regularly invoked to condemn repressive practices and ideals, repression being conceived of as an environment that deprives one of strength (TB) or of flexibility and spontaneity (cancer). Modern disease metaphors specify an ideal of society's well-being, analogized to physical health, that is as frequently anti-political as it is a call for a new political order.

Order is the oldest concern of political philosophy, and if it is plausible to compare the polis to an organism, then it is plausible to compare civil disorder to an illness. The classical formulations which analogize a political disorder to an illness – from Plato to, say, Hobbes – presuppose the classical medical (and political) idea of balance. Illness comes from imbalance. Treatment is aimed at restoring the right balance – in political terms, the right hierarchy. The prognosis is always, in principle, optimistic. Society, by definition, never catches a fatal disease.

When a disease image is used by Machiavelli, the presumption is that the disease can be cured. 'Consumption,' he wrote,

in the commencement is easy to cure, and difficult to understand; but when it has neither been discovered in due time, nor treated upon a proper principle, it becomes easy to understand, and difficult to cure. The same thing happens in state affairs, by foreseeing them at a distance, which is only done by men of talents, the evils which might arise from them are soon cured; but when, from want of foresight, they are suffered to increase to such a height that they are perceptible to everyone, there is no longer any remedy.

77

Machiavelli invokes TB as a disease whose progress can be cut off, if it is detected at an early stage (when its symptoms are barely visible). Given proper foresight, the course of a disease is not irreversible; the same for disturbances in the body politic. Machiavelli offers an illness metaphor that is not so much about society as about statecraft (conceived as a therapeutic art): as prudence is needed to control serious diseases, so foresight is needed to control social crises. It is a metaphor about foresight, and a call to foresight.

In political philosophy's great tradition, the analogy between disease and civil disorder is proposed to encourage rulers to pursue a more rational policy. 'Although nothing can be immortal, which mortals make,' Hobbes wrote,

> yet, if men had the use of reason they pretend to, their Commonwealths might be secured, at least, from perishing by internal diseases ... Therefore when they come to be dissolved, not by externall violence, but intestine disorder, the fault is not in men, as they are the *Matter*; but as they are the *Makers*, and orderers of them.

Hobbes's view is anything but fatalistic. Rulers have the responsibility and the ability (through reason) to control disorder. For Hobbes, murder ('externall violence') is the only 'natural' way for a society or institution to die. To perish from internal disorder – analogized to a disease – is suicide, something quite preventable; an act of will, or rather a failure of will (that is, of reason).

The disease metaphor was used in political philosophy

to reinforce the call for a rational response. Machiavelli and Hobbes fixed on one part of medical wisdom, the importance of cutting off serious disease early, while it is relatively easy to control. The disease metaphor could also be used to encourage rulers to another kind of foresight. In 1708, Lord Shaftesbury wrote:

> There are certain humours in mankind which of necessity must have vent. The human mind and body are both of them naturally subject to commotions ... as there are strange ferments in the blood, which in many bodies occasion an extra-ordinary discharge ... Should physicians endeavour absolutely to allay those ferments of the body, and strike in the humours which discover themselves in such eruptions, they might, instead of making a cure, bid fair perhaps to raise a plague, and turn a spring-ague or an autumn-surfeit into an epidemical malignant fever. They are certainly as ill physicians in the body politic who would needs be tampering with these mental eruptions, and, under the specious pretence of healing this itch of superstition and saving souls from the contagion of enthusiasm, should set all nature in an uproar, and turn a few innocent carbuncles into an inflammation and mortal gangrene.

Shaftesbury's point is that it is rational to tolerate a certain amount of irrationality ('superstition,' 'enthusiasm'), and that stern repressive measures are likely to aggravate disorder rather than cure it, turning a nuisance into a disaster. The body politic should not be overmedicalized; a remedy should not be sought for every disorder.

For Machiavelli, foresight; for Hobbes, reason; for

Shaftesbury, tolerance – these are all ideas of how proper statecraft, conceived on a medical analogy, can prevent a fatal disorder. Society is presumed to be in basically good health; disease (disorder) is, in principle, always manageable.

In the modern period, the use of disease imagery in political rhetoric implies other, less lenient assumptions. The modern idea of revolution, based on an estimate of the unremitting bleakness of the existing political situation, shattered the old, optimistic use of disease metaphors. John Adams' wrote in his diary, in December 1772:

> The Prospect before me ... is very gloomy. My Country is in deep Distress, and has very little Ground of Hope ... The Body of the People seem to be worn out, by struggling, and Venality, Servility and Prostitution, eat and spread like a Cancer.

Political events started commonly to be defined as being unprecedented, radical; and eventually both civil disturbances and wars come to be understood as, really, revolutions. As might be expected, it was not with the American but with the French Revolution that disease metaphors in the modern sense came into their own – particularly in the conservative response to the French Revolution. In *Reflections on the Revolution in France* (1790), Edmund Burke contrasted older wars and civil disturbances with this one, which he considered to have a totally new character. Before, no matter what the disaster, 'the organs ... of the state, however shattered, existed.' But, he addressed the French, 'your present confusion, like a palsy, has attacked the fountain of life itself.'

As classical theories of the polis have gone the way of the theories of the four humors, so a modern idea of politics has been complemented by a modern idea of disease. Disease equals death. Burke invoked palsy (and 'the living ulcer of a corroding memory'). The emphasis was soon to be on diseases that are loathsome and fatal. Such diseases are not to be managed or treated; they are to be attacked. In Hugo's novel about the French Revolution, *Quatre-vingt-treize* (1874), the revolutionary Gauvain, condemned to the guillotine, absolves the Revolution with all its bloodshed, including his own imminent execution,

> because it is a storm. A storm always knows what it is doing ... Civilization was in the grip of plague; this gale comes to the rescue. Perhaps it is not selective enough. Can it act otherwise? It is entrusted with the arduous task of sweeping away disease! In face of the horrible infection, I understand the fury of the blast.

It is hardly the last time that revolutionary violence would be justified on the grounds that society has a radical, horrible illness. The melodramatics of the disease metaphor in modern political discourse assume a punitive notion: of the disease not as a punishment but as a sign of evil, something to be punished.

Modern totalitarian movements, whether of the right

or of the left, have been peculiarly – and revealingly – inclined to use disease imagery. The Nazis declared that someone of mixed 'racial' origin was like a syphilitic. European Jewry was repeatedly analogized to syphilis, and to a cancer that must be excised. Disease metaphors were a staple of Bolshevik polemics, and Trotsky, the most gifted of all communist polemicists, used them with the greatest profusion – particularly after his banishment from the Soviet Union in 1929. Stalinism was called a cholera, a syphilis, and a cancer.* To use only fatal diseases for imagery in politics gives the metaphor a much more pointed character. Now, to liken a political event or situation to an illness is to impute guilt, to prescribe punishment.

This is particularly true of the use of cancer as a

---

* Cf. Isaac Deutscher, *The Prophet Outcast: Trotsky, 1929–1940* (1963): '"Certain measures," Trotsky wrote to [Philip] Rahv [on March 21, 1938], "are necessary for a struggle against incorrect theory, and others for fighting a cholera epidemic. Stalin is incomparably nearer to cholera than to a false theory. The struggle must be intense, truculent, merciless. An element of 'fanaticism' ... is salutary."' And: 'Trotsky spoke of the "syphilis of Stalinism" or of the "cancer that must be burned out of the labour movement with a hot iron." ...'

Notably, Solzhenitsyn's *Cancer Ward* contains virtually no uses of cancer as a metaphor – for Stalinism, or for anything else. Solzhenitsyn was not misrepresenting his novel when, hoping to get it published in the Soviet Union, he told the Board of the Union of Writers in 1967 that the title was not 'some kind of symbol,' as was being charged, and that 'the subject is specifically and literally cancer.'

metaphor. It amounts to saying, first of all, that the event or situation is unqualifiedly and unredeemably wicked. It enormously ups the ante. Hitler, in his first political tract, an anti-Semitic diatribe written in September 1919, accused the Jews of producing 'a racial tuberculosis among nations.'* Tuberculosis still retained its prestige as the overdetermined, culpable illness of the nineteenth century. (Recall Hugo's comparison of monasticism with TB.) But the Nazis quickly modernized their rhetoric, and indeed the imagery of cancer was far more apt for their purposes. As was said in speeches about 'the Jewish problem' throughout the 1930s, to treat a cancer, one must cut out much of the healthy tissue around it. The imagery of cancer for the Nazis prescribes 'radical' treatment, in contrast to the 'soft' treatment thought appropriate for TB – the difference between sanatoria (that is, exile) and surgery (that is, crematoria). (The Jews were also identified with, and became a metaphor for, city life – with Nazi rhetoric

* '[The Jew's] power is the power of money which in the form of interest effortlessly and interminably multiples itself in his hands and forces upon nations that most dangerous of yokes ... Everything which makes men strive for higher things, whether religion, socialism, or democracy, is for him only a means to an end, to the satisfaction of a lust for money and domination. His activities produce a racial tuberculosis among nations ...' A late-nineteenth-century precursor of Nazi ideology, Julius Langbehn, called the Jews 'only a passing pest and cholera.' But in Hitler's TB image there is already something easily transferred to cancer: the idea that Jewish power 'effortlessly and interminably multiplies.'

echoing all the Romantic clichés about cities as a debilitating, merely cerebral, morally contaminated, unhealthy environment.)

To describe a phenomenon as a cancer is an incitement to violence. The use of cancer in political discourse encourages fatalism and justifies 'severe' measures – as well as strongly reinforcing the widespread notion that the disease is necessarily fatal. The concept of disease is never innocent. But it could be argued that the cancer metaphors are in themselves implicitly genocidal. No specific political view seems to have a monopoly on this metaphor. Trotsky called Stalinism the cancer of Marxism; in China in the last year, the Gang of Four have become, among other things, 'the cancer of China.' John Dean explained Watergate to Nixon: 'We have a cancer within – close to the Presidency – that's growing.' The standard metaphor of Arab polemics – heard by Israelis on the radio every day for the last twenty years – is that Israel is 'a cancer in the heart of the Arab world' or 'the cancer of the Middle East,' and an officer with the Christian Lebanese rightist forces besieging the Palestine refugee camp of Tal Zaatar in August 1976 called the camp 'a cancer in the Lebanese body.' The cancer metaphor seems hard to resist for those who wish to register indignation. Thus, Neal Ascherson wrote in 1969 that the Slansky Affair 'was – is – a huge cancer in the body of the Czechoslovak state and nation'; Simon Leys, in *Chinese Shadows*, speaks of 'the Maoist cancer that is gnawing away at the face of China'; D. H. Lawrence called masturbation 'the deepest and most dangerous cancer of our civilization'; and I once wrote, in the heat of despair over America's war on Vietnam, that 'the white race is the cancer of human history.'

But how to be morally severe in the late twentieth century? How, when there is so much to be severe about; how, when we have a sense of evil but no longer the religious or philosophical language to talk intelligently about evil. Trying to comprehend 'radical' or 'absolute' evil, we search for adequate metaphors. But the modern disease metaphors are all cheap shots. The people who have the real disease are also hardly helped by hearing their disease's name constantly being dropped as the epitome of evil. Only in the most limited sense is any historical event or problem like an illness. And the cancer metaphor is particularly crass. It is invariably an encouragement to simplify what is complex and an invitation to self-righteousness, if not to fanaticism.

It is instructive to compare the image of cancer with that of gangrene. With some of the same metaphoric properties as cancer – it starts from nothing; it spreads; it is disgusting – gangrene would seem to be laden with everything a polemicist would want. Indeed, it was used in one important moral polemic – against the French use of torture in Algeria in the 1950s; the title of the famous book exposing that torture was called *La Gangrène*. But there is a large difference between the cancer and the gangrene metaphors. First, causality is clear with gangrene. It is external (gangrene can develop from a scratch); cancer is understood as mysterious, a disease with multiple causes, internal as well as external. Second, gangrene is not as all-encompassing a disaster. It leads often to amputation, less often to death; cancer is presumed to lead to death in most cases. Not gangrene – and not the plague (despite the notable attempts by writers as different as Artaud, Reich, and Camus to impose that as a metaphor for the dismal and the disastrous) – but cancer remains the most radical of disease metaphors. And just because it is so radical, it is particularly tendentious – a good metaphor for paranoids, for those who need to turn campaigns into crusades, for the fatalistic (cancer = death), and for those under the spell of a historical revolutionary optimism (the idea that only the most radical changes are desirable). As long as so much militaristic hyperbole attaches to the description and treatment of cancer, it is a particularly unapt metaphor for the peaceloving.

It is, of course, likely that the language about cancer will evolve in the coming years. It must change, decisively, when the disease is finally understood and the rate of cure becomes much higher. It is already changing, with the development of new forms of treatment. As chemotherapy is more and more supplanting radiation in the treatment of cancer patients, an effective form of treatment (already a supplementary treatment of proven use) seems likely to be found in some kind of immunotherapy. Concepts have started to shift in certain medical circles, where doctors are concentrating on the steep buildup of the body's immunological responses to cancer. As the language of treatment evolves from military metaphors of aggressive warfare to metaphors featuring the body's 'natural defenses' (what is called the 'immunodefensive system' can also – to break entirely with the military metaphor – be called the body's 'immune competence'), cancer will be partly de-mythicized; and it may then be possible to compare something to a cancer without implying either a fatalistic diagnosis or a rousing call to fight by any means whatever a lethal, insidious enemy. Then perhaps it will be morally permissible, as it is not now, to use cancer as a metaphor.

But at that time, perhaps nobody will want any longer to compare anything awful to cancer. Since the interest of the metaphor is precisely that it refers to a disease so overlaid with mystification, so charged with the fantasy of inescapable fatality. Since our views about cancer, and the metaphors we have imposed on it, are so much a vehicle for the large insufficiencies of this culture, for our shallow attitude toward death, for our anxieties about feeling, for our reckless improvident responses to our real 'problems of growth,' for our inability to construct an advanced industrial society which properly regulates consumption, and for our justified fears of the increasingly violent course of history. The cancer metaphor will be made obsolete, I would predict, long before the problems it has reflected so persuasively will be resolved.

AIDS AND ITS METAPHORS

Rereading *Illness as Metaphor* now, I thought:

Chapter One

By metaphor I meant nothing more or less than the earliest and most succinct definition I know, which is Aristotle's in his *Poetics* (1457b). 'Metaphor,' Aristotle wrote, 'consists in giving the thing a name that belongs to something else.' Saying a thing is or is like something-it-is-not is a mental operation as old as philosophy and poetry, and the spawning ground of most kinds of understanding, including scientific understanding, and expressiveness. (To acknowledge which I prefaced the polemic against metaphors of illness I wrote ten years ago with a brief, hectic flourish of metaphor, in mock exorcism of the seductiveness of metaphorical thinking.) Of course, one cannot think without metaphors. But that does not mean there aren't some metaphors we might well abstain from or try to retire. As, of course, all thinking is interpretation. But that does not mean it isn't sometimes correct to be 'against' interpretation.

Take, for instance, a tenacious metaphor that has

shaped (and obscured the understanding of) so much of the political life of this century, the one that distributes and polarizes, attitudes and social movements according to their relation to a 'left' and a 'right.' The terms are usually traced back to the French Revolution, to the seating arrangements of the National Assembly in 1789, when republicans and radicals sat to the presiding officer's left and monarchists and conservatives sat to the right. But historical memory alone can't account for the startling longevity of this metaphor. It seems more likely that its persistence in discourse about politics to this day comes from a felt aptness to the modern, secular imagination of metaphors drawn from the body's orientation in space – left and right, top and bottom, forward and backward – for describing social conflict, a metaphoric practice that did add something new to the perennial description of society as a kind of body, a well-disciplined body ruled by a 'head.' This has been the dominant metaphor for the polity since Plato and Aristotle, perhaps because of its usefulness in justifying repression. Even more than comparing society to a family, comparing it to a body makes an authoritarian ordering of society seem inevitable, immutable.

Rudolf Virchow, the founder of cellular pathology, furnishes one of the rare scientifically significant examples of the reverse procedure, using political metaphors to talk about the body. In the biological controversies of the 1850s, it was the metaphor of the liberal state that Virchow found useful in advancing his theory of the cell as the fundamental unit of life. However complex their structures, organisms are, first of all, simply 'multicellular' – multicitizened, as it were; the body is a 'republic' or 'unified commonwealth.' Among scientist-rhetoricians Virchow was a maverick, not least because of the politics of his metaphors, which, by mid-nineteenth-century standards, are antiauthoritarian. But likening the body to a society, liberal or not, is less common than comparisons to other complex, integrated systems, such as a machine or an economic enterprise.

At the beginning of Western medicine, in Greece, important metaphors for the unity of the body were adapted from the arts. One such metaphor, harmony, was singled out for scorn several centuries later by Lucretius, who argued that it could not do justice to the fact that the body consists of essential and unessential organs, or even to the body's materiality: that is, to death. Here are the closing lines of Lucretius' dismissal of the musical metaphor – the earliest attack I know on metaphoric thinking about illness and health:

> Not all the organs, you must realize,
> Are equally important nor does health
> Depend on all alike, but there are some –
> The seeds of breathing, warm vitality –
> Whereby we are kept alive; when these are gone
> Life leaves our dying members. So, since mind
> And spirit are by nature part of man,
> Let the musicians keep that term brought down
> To them from lofty Helicon – or maybe
> They found it somewhere else, made it apply
> To something hitherto nameless in their craft –

I speak of *harmony*. Whatever it is,
Give it back to the musicians.

De Rerum Natura III, 124–35
trans. Rolfe Humphries

A history of metaphoric thinking about the body on this potent level of generality would include many images drawn from other arts and technology, notably architecture. Some metaphors are anti-explanatory, like the sermonizing, and poetic, notion enunciated by Saint Paul of the body as a temple. Some have considerable scientific resonance, such as the notion of the body as a factory, an image of the body's functioning under the sign of health, and of the body as a fortress, an image of the body that features catastrophe.

The fortress image has a long prescientific genealogy, with illness itself a metaphor for mortality, for human frailty and vulnerability. John Donne in his great cycle of prose arias on illness, *Devotions upon Emergent Occasions* (1627), written when he thought he was dying, describes illness as an enemy that invades, that lays siege to the body-fortress:

> We study Health, and we deliberate upon our meats, and drink, and ayre, and exercises, and we hew and wee polish every stone, that goes to that building; and so our Health is a long and a regular work; But in a minute a Canon batters all, overthrowes all, demolishes all; a Sicknes unprevented for all our diligence, unsuspected for all our curiositie . . .

Some parts are more fragile than others: Donne speaks

of the brain and the liver being able to endure the siege of an 'unnatural' or 'rebellious' fever that 'will blow up the heart, like a mine, in a minute.' In Donne's images, it is the illness that invades. Modern medical thinking could be said to begin when the gross military metaphor becomes specific, which can only happen with the advent of a new kind of scrutiny, represented in Virchow's cellular pathology, and a more precise understanding that illnesses were caused by specific identifiable, visible (with the aid of a microscope) organisms. It was when the invader was seen not as the illness but as the micro-organism that causes the illness that medicine really began to be effective, and the military metaphors took on new credibility and precision. Since then, military metaphors have more and more come to infuse all aspects of the description of the medical situation. Disease is seen as an invasion of alien organisms, to which the body responds by its own military operations, such as the mobilizing of immunological 'defenses,' and medicine is 'aggressive,' as in the language of most chemotherapies.

The grosser metaphor survives in public health education, where disease is regularly described as invading the society, and efforts to reduce mortality from a given disease are called a fight, a struggle, a war. Military metaphors became prominent early in the century, in campaigns mounted during World War I to educate people about syphilis, and after the war about tuberculosis. One example, from the campaign against tuberculosis conducted in Italy in the 1920s, is a poster called 'Guerre alle Mosche' (War against Flies), which illustrates the lethal effects of fly-borne diseases. The flies themselves are shown as enemy aircraft dropping bombs of death on an innocent population. The bombs have inscriptions. One says 'Microbi,' microbes. Another says, 'Germi della tisi,' the germs of tuberculosis. Another simply says 'Malattia,' illness. A skeleton clad in a hooded black cloak rides the foremost fly as passenger or pilot. In another poster, 'With These Weapons We Will Conquer Tuberculosis,' the figure of death is shown pinned to the wall by drawn swords, each of which bears an inscription that names a measure for combating tuberculosis. 'Cleanliness' is written on one blade. 'Sun' on another. 'Air.' 'Rest.' 'Proper food.' 'Hygiene.' (Of course, none of these weapons was of any significance. What conquers – that is, cures – tuberculosis is antibiotics, which were not discovered until some twenty years later, in the 1940s.)

Where once it was the physician who waged *bellum contra morbum*, the war against disease, now it's the whole society. Indeed, the transformation of war-making into an occasion for mass ideological mobilization has made the notion of war useful as a metaphor for all sorts of ameliorative campaigns whose goals are cast as the defeat of an 'enemy.' We have had wars against poverty, now replaced by 'the war on drugs,' as well as wars against specific diseases, such as cancer. Abuse of the military metaphor may be inevitable in a capitalist society, a society that increasingly restricts the scope and credibility of appeals to ethical principle, in which it is thought foolish not to subject one's actions to the calculus of self-interest and profitability. War-making is one of the few activities that people are not supposed to view 'realistically'; that is, with an eye to expense and practical outcome. In all-out war, expenditure is all-out, unprudent – war being defined as an emergency in which no sacrifice is excessive. But the wars against diseases are not just calls for more zeal, and more money to be spent on research. The metaphor implements the way particularly dreaded diseases are envisaged as an alien 'other,' as enemies are in modern war; and the move from the demonization of the illness to the attribution of fault to the patient is an inevitable one, no matter if patients are thought of as victims. Victims suggest innocence. And innocence, by the inexorable logic that governs all relational terms, suggests guilt.

Military metaphors contribute to the stigmatizing of certain illnesses and, by extension, of those who are ill. It was the discovery of the stigmatization of people who have cancer that led me to write *Illness as Metaphor*.

Twelve years ago, when I became a cancer patient, what particularly enraged me – and distracted me from my own terror and despair at my doctors' gloomy prognosis – was seeing how much the very reputation of this illness added to the suffering of those who have it. Many fellow patients with whom I talked during my initial hospitalizations, like others I was to meet during the subsequent two and a half years that I received chemotherapy as an outpatient in several hospitals here and in

France, evinced disgust at their disease and a kind of shame. They seemed to be in the grip of fantasies about their illness by which I was quite unseduced. And it occurred to me that some of these notions were the converse of now thoroughly discredited beliefs about tuberculosis. As tuberculosis had been often regarded sentimentally, as an enhancement of identity, cancer was regarded with irrational revulsion, as a diminution of the self. There were also similar fictions of responsibility and of a characterological predisposition to the illness: cancer is regarded as a disease to which the psychically defeated, the inexpressive, the repressed – especially those who have repressed anger or sexual feelings – are particularly prone, as tuberculosis was regarded throughout the nineteenth and early twentieth centuries (indeed, until it was discovered how to cure it) as a disease apt to strike the hypersensitive, the talented, the passionate.

These parallels – between myths about tuberculosis to which we can all feel superior now, and superstitions about cancer still given credence by many cancer patients and their families – gave me the main strategy of a little book I decided to write about the mystifications surrounding cancer. I didn't think it would be useful – and I wanted to be useful – to tell yet one more story in the first person of how someone learned that she or he had cancer, wept, struggled, was comforted, suffered, took courage . . . though mine was also that story. A narrative, it seemed to me, would be less useful than an idea. For narrative pleasure I would appeal to other writers; and although more examples from literature immediately came to mind for the glamorous disease, tuberculosis, I found the diagnosis of cancer as a disease of those who have not really lived in such books as Tolstoy's *The Death of Ivan Ilyich*, Arnold Bennett's *Riceyman Steps*, and Bernanos's *The Diary of a Country Priest*.

And so I wrote my book, wrote it very quickly, spurred by evangelical zeal as well as anxiety about how much time I had left to do any living or writing in. My aim was to alleviate unnecessary suffering – exactly as Nietzsche formulated it, in a passage in *Daybreak* that I came across recently:

> *Thinking about illness!* – To calm the imagination of the invalid, so that at least he should not, as hitherto, have to suffer more from thinking about his illness than from the illness itself – that, I think, would be something! It would be a great deal!

The purpose of my book was to calm the imagination, not to incite it. Not to confer meaning, which is the traditional purpose of literary endeavor, but to deprive something of meaning: to apply that quixotic, highly polemical strategy, 'against interpretation,' to the real world this time. To the body. My purpose was, above all, practical. For it was my doleful observation, repeated again and again, that the metaphoric trappings that deform the experience of having cancer have very real consequences: they inhibit people from seeking treatment early enough, or from making a greater effort to get competent treatment. The metaphors and myths, I was convinced, kill. (For instance, they make people

99

irrationally fearful of effective measures such as chemo-therapy, and foster credence in thoroughly useless remedies such as diets and psychotherapy.) I wanted to offer other people who were ill and those who care for them an instrument to dissolve these metaphors, these inhibitions. I hoped to persuade terrified people who were ill to consult doctors, or to change their incompe-tent doctors for competent ones, who would give them proper care. To regard cancer as if it were just a disease – a very serious one, but just a disease. Not a curse, not a punishment, not an embarrassment. Without 'meaning.' And not necessarily a death sentence (one of the mystifica-tions is that cancer = death). *Illness as Metaphor* is not just a polemic, it is an exhortation. I was saying: Get the doctors to tell you the truth; be an informed, active patient; find yourself good treatment, because good treatment does exist (amid the widespread ineptitude). Although *the* remedy does not exist, more than half of all cases can be cured by existing methods of treatment.

In the decade since I wrote *Illness as Metaphor* – and was cured of my own cancer, confounding my doctors' pessimism – attitudes about cancer have evolved. Getting cancer is not quite as much of a stigma, a creator of 'spoiled identity' (to use Erving Goffman's expression). The word cancer is uttered more freely, and people are not often described anymore in obituaries as dying of a 'very long illness.' Although European and Japanese doctors still regularly impart a cancer diagnosis first to the family, and often counsel concealing it from the patient, American doctors have virtually abandoned this policy; indeed, a brutal announcement to the patient is now common. The new candor about cancer is part of the same obligatory candor (or lack of decorum) that brings us diagrams of the rectal-colon or genito-urinary tract ailments of our national leaders on television and on the front pages of newspapers – more and more it is precisely a virtue in our society to speak of what is supposed *not* to be named. The change can also be explained by the doctors' fear of lawsuits in a litigious society. And not least among the reasons that cancer is now treated less phobically, certainly with less secrecy, than a decade ago is that it is no longer the most feared disease. In recent years some of the onus of cancer has been lifted by the emergence of a disease whose charge of stigmatization, whose capacity to create spoiled identity, is far greater. It seems that societies need to have one illness which becomes identified with evil, and attaches blame to its 'victims,' but it is hard to be obsessed with more than one.

Chapter Two

Just as one might predict for a disease that is not yet
fully understood as well as extremely recalcitrant to treatment, the advent of this terrifying new disease, new at
least in its epidemic form, has provided a large-scale
occasion for the metaphorizing of illness.

Strictly speaking, AIDS – acquired immune deficiency syndrome – is not the name of an illness at all. It
is the name of a medical condition, whose consequences
are a spectrum of illnesses. In contrast to syphilis and
cancer, which provide prototypes for most of the images
and metaphors attached to AIDS, the very definition of
AIDS requires the presence of other illnesses, so-called
opportunistic infections and malignancies. But though
not in *that* sense a single disease, AIDS lends itself to
being regarded as one – in part because, unlike cancer
and like syphilis, it is thought to have a single cause.

AIDS has a dual metaphoric genealogy. As a micro-
process, it is described as cancer is: an invasion. When

the focus is transmission of the disease, an older meta-phor, reminiscent of syphilis, is invoked: pollution. (One gets it from the blood or sexual fluids of infected people or from contaminated blood products.) But the military metaphors used to describe AIDS have a somewhat different focus from those used in describing cancer. With cancer, the metaphor scants the issue of causality (still a murky topic in cancer research) and picks up at the point at which rogue cells inside the body mutate, eventually moving out from an original site or organ to overrun other organs or systems – a domestic subversion. In the description of AIDS the enemy is what causes the disease, an infectious agent that comes from the outside:

> The invader is tiny, about one sixteen-thousandth the size of the head of a pin ... Scouts of the body's immune system, large cells called macrophages, sense the presence of the diminutive foreigner and promptly alert the immune system. It begins to mobilize an array of cells that, among other things, produce antibodies to deal with the threat. Single-mindedly, the AIDS virus ignores many of the blood cells in its path, evades the rapidly advancing defenders and homes in on the master coordinator of the immune system, a helper T cell ...

This is the language of political paranoia, with its charac-teristic distrust of a pluralistic world. A defense system consisting of cells 'that, among other things, produce antibodies to deal with the threat' is, predictably, no match for an invader who advances 'single-mindedly.' And the science-fiction flavor, already present in cancer talk, is even more pungent in accounts of AIDS – this one comes from *Time* magazine in late 1986 – with infection described like the high-tech warfare for which we are being prepared (and inured) by the fantasies of our leaders and by video entertainments. In the era of Star Wars and Space Invaders, AIDS has proved an ideally comprehensible illness:

> On the surface of that cell, it finds a receptor into which one of its envelope proteins fits perfectly, like a key into a lock. Docking with the cell, the virus penetrates the cell membrane and is stripped of its protective shell in the process . . .

Next the invader takes up permanent residence, by a form of alien takeover familiar in science-fiction narratives. The body's own cells *become* the invader. With the help of an enzyme the virus carries with it,

> the naked AIDS virus converts its RNA into . . . DNA, the master molecule of life. The molecule then penetrates the cell nucleus, inserts itself into a chromosome and takes over part of the cellular machinery, directing it to produce more AIDS viruses. Eventually, overcome by its alien product, the cell swells and dies, releasing a flood of new viruses to attack other cells . . .

As viruses attack other cells, runs the metaphor, so 'a host of opportunistic diseases, normally warded off by a healthy immune system, attacks the body,' whose integrity and vigor have been sapped by the sheer replication of 'alien product' that follows the collapse of its immunological defenses. 'Gradually weakened by the onslaught, the AIDS victim dies, sometimes in months, but almost always within a few years of the first symptoms.' Those who have not already succumbed are described as 'under assault, showing the telltale symptoms of the disease,' while millions of others 'harbor the virus, vulnerable at any time to a final, all-out attack.'

Cancer makes cells proliferate; in AIDS, cells die. Even as this original model of AIDS (the mirror image of leukemia) has been altered, descriptions of how the virus does its work continue to echo the way the illness is perceived as infiltrating the society. 'AIDS Virus Found to Hide in Cells, Eluding Detection by Normal Tests' was the headline of a recent front-page story in *The New York Times* announcing the discovery that the virus can 'lurk' for years in the macrophages – disrupting their disease-fighting function without killing them, 'even when the macrophages are filled almost to bursting with virus,' and without producing antibodies, the chemicals the body makes in response to 'invading agents' and whose presence has been regarded as an infallible marker of the syndrome.* That the virus isn't lethal for

* The larger role assigned to the macrophages – 'to serve as a reservoir for the AIDS virus because the virus multiplies in them but does not kill them, as it kills T-4 cells' – is said to explain the not uncommon difficulty of finding infected T-4 lymphocytes in patients who have antibodies to the virus and symptoms of AIDS. (It is still assumed that antibodies will develop once the virus spreads to these 'key target' cells.) Evidence of presently infected populations of cells has been as puzzlingly limited or uneven as the evidence of infection in the populations of human societies –

all the cells where it takes up residence, as is now thought, only increases the illness-foe's reputation for wiliness and invincibility.

What makes the viral assault so terrifying is that contamination, and therefore vulnerability, is understood as permanent. Even if someone infected were never to develop any symptoms – that is, the infection remained, or could by medical intervention be rendered, inactive – the viral enemy would be forever within. In fact, so it is believed, it is just a matter of time before something awakens ('triggers') it, before the appearance of 'the telltale symptoms.' Like syphilis, known to generations of doctors as 'the great masquerader,' AIDS is a clinical construction, an inference. It takes its identity from the presence of *some* among a long, and lengthening, roster of symptoms (no one has everything that AIDS could be), symptoms which 'mean' that what the patient has is this illness. The construction of the illness rests on the invention not only of AIDS as a clinical entity but of a kind of junior AIDS, called AIDS-related complex (ARC), to which people are assigned if they show 'early' and often intermittent symptoms of immunological deficit such as fevers, weight loss, fungal infections, and

---

puzzling, because of the conviction that the disease is everywhere, and must spread. 'Doctors have estimated that as few as one in a million T-4 cells are infected, which led some to ask where the virus hides . . .' Another resonant speculation, reported in the same article (*The New York Times*, June 7, 1988): 'Infected macrophages can transmit the virus to other cells, possibly by touching the cells.'

swollen lymph glands. AIDS is progressive, a disease of time. Once a certain density of symptoms is attained, the course of the illness can be swift, and brings atrocious suffering. Besides the commonest 'presenting' illnesses (some hitherto unusual, at least in a fatal form, such as a rare skin cancer and a rare form of pneumonia), a plethora of disabling, disfiguring, and humiliating symptoms make the AIDS patient steadily more infirm, helpless, and unable to control or take care of basic functions and needs.

The sense in which AIDS is a slow disease makes it more like syphilis, which is characterized in terms of 'stages,' than like cancer. Thinking in terms of 'stages' is essential to discourse about AIDS. Syphilis in its most dreaded form is 'tertiary syphilis,' syphilis in its third stage. What is called AIDS is generally understood as the last of three stages – the first of which is infection with a human immunodeficiency virus (HIV) and early evidence of inroads on the immune system – with a long latency period between infection and the onset of the 'telltale' symptoms. (Apparently not as long as syphilis, in which the latency period between secondary and tertiary illness might be decades. But it is worth noting that when syphilis first appeared in epidemic form in Europe at the end of the fifteenth century, it was a rapid disease, of an unexplained virulence that is unknown today, in which death often occurred in the second stage, sometimes within months or a few years.) Cancer *grows* slowly: it is not thought to be, for a long time, latent. (A convincing account of a process in terms of 'stages' seems invariably to include the notion of a normative delay or halt in the process, such as is supplied by the notion of latency.) True, a cancer is 'staged.' This is a principal tool of diagnosis, which means classifying it according to its gravity, determining how 'advanced' it is. But it is mostly a spatial notion: that the cancer advances through the body, traveling or migrating along predictable routes. Cancer is first of all a disease of the body's geography, in contrast to syphilis and AIDS, whose definition depends on constructing a temporal sequence of stages.

Syphilis is an affliction that didn't have to run its ghastly full course, to paresis (as it did for Baudelaire and Maupassant and Jules de Goncourt), and could and often did remain at the stage of nuisance, indignity (as it did for Flaubert). The scourge was also a cliché, as Flaubert himself observed. 'SYPHILIS. Everybody has it, more or less' reads one entry in the *Dictionary of Accepted Opinions*, his treasury of mid-nineteenth-century platitudes. And syphilis did manage to acquire a darkly positive association in late-nineteenth- and early-twentieth-century Europe, when a link was made between syphilis and heightened ('feverish') mental activity that parallels the connection made since the era of the Romantic writers between pulmonary tuberculosis and heightened emotional activity. As if in honor of all the notable writers and artists who ended their lives in syphilitic witlessness, it came to be believed that the brain lesions of neurosyphilis might actually inspire original thought or art. Thomas Mann, whose fiction is a storehouse of early-twentieth-century disease myths, makes this notion of syphilis as muse central to his *Doctor Faustus*, with its protagonist a great composer whose voluntarily contracted syphilis – the Devil guarantees that the infection will be limited to the central nervous system – confers on him twenty-four years of incandescent creativity. E. M. Cioran recalls how, in Romania in the late 1920s, syphilis-envy figured in his adolescent expectations of literary glory: he would discover that he had contracted syphilis, be rewarded with several hyperproductive years of genius, then collapse into madness. This romanticizing of the dementia characteristic of neurosyphilis was the forerunner of the much more persistent fantasy in this century about mental illness as a source of artistic creativity or spiritual originality. But with AIDS – though dementia is also a common, late symptom – no compensatory mythology has arisen, or seems likely to arise. AIDS, like cancer, does not allow romanticizing or sentimentalizing, perhaps because its association with death is too powerful. In Krzysztof Zanussi's film *Spiral* (1978), the most truthful account I know of anger at dying, the protagonist's illness is never specified; therefore, it *has* to be cancer. For several generations now, the generic idea of death has been a death from cancer, and a cancer death is experienced as a generic defeat. Now the generic rebuke to life and to hope is AIDS.

Chapter Three

Because of countless metaphoric flourishes that have made cancer synonymous with evil, having cancer has been experienced by many as shameful, therefore something to conceal, and also unjust, a betrayal by one's body. Why me? the cancer patient exclaims bitterly. With AIDS, the shame is linked to an imputation of guilt; and the scandal is not at all obscure. Few wonder, Why me? Most people outside of sub-Saharan Africa who have AIDS know (or think they know) how they got it. It is not a mysterious affliction that seems to strike at random. Indeed, to get AIDS is precisely to be revealed, in the majority of cases so far, as a member of a certain 'risk group,' a community of pariahs. The illness flushes out an identity that might have remained hidden from neighbors, jobmates, family, friends. It also confirms an identity and, among the risk group in the United States most severely affected in the beginning, homosexual men, has been a creator of community as well as an experience that isolates the ill and exposes them to harassment and persecution.

Getting cancer, too, is sometimes understood as the fault of someone who has indulged in 'unsafe' behavior – the alcoholic with cancer of the esophagus, the smoker with lung cancer: punishment for living unhealthy lives. (In contrast to those obliged to perform unsafe occupations, like the worker in a petrochemical factory who gets bladder cancer.) More and more linkages are sought between primary organs or systems and specific practices that people are invited to repudiate, as in recent speculation associating colon cancer and breast cancer with diets rich in animal fats. But the unsafe habits associated with cancer, among other illnesses – even heart disease, hitherto little culpabilized, is now largely viewed as the price one pays for excesses of diet and 'life-style' – are the result of a weakness of the will or a lack of prudence, or of addiction to legal (albeit very dangerous) chemicals. The unsafe behavior that produces AIDS is judged to be more than just weakness. It is indulgence, delinquency – addictions to chemicals that are illegal and to sex regarded as deviant.

The sexual transmission of this illness, considered by most people as a calamity one brings on oneself, is judged more harshly than other means – especially since AIDS is understood as a disease not only of sexual excess but of perversity. (I am thinking, of course, of the United States, where people are currently being told that heterosexual transmission is extremely rare, and unlikely – as if Africa did not exist.) An infectious disease whose principal means of transmission is sexual necessarily puts at greater risk those who are sexually more active – and is easy to view as a punishment for that activity. True of syphilis, this is even truer of AIDS, since not just promiscuity but a specific sexual 'practice' regarded as unnatural is named as more endangering. Getting the disease through a sexual practice is thought to be more willful, therefore deserves more blame. Addicts who get the illness by sharing contaminated needles are seen as committing (or completing) a kind of inadvertent suicide. Promiscuous homosexual men practicing their vehement sexual customs under the illusory conviction, fostered by medical ideology with its cure-all antibiotics, of the relative innocuousness of all sexually transmitted diseases, could be viewed as dedicated hedonists – though it's now clear that their behavior was no less suicidal. Those like hemophiliacs and blood-transfusion recipients, who cannot by any stretch of the blaming faculty be considered responsible for their illness, may be as ruthlessly ostracized by frightened people, and potentially represent a greater threat because, unlike the already stigmatized, they are not as easy to identify.

Infectious diseases to which sexual fault is attached always inspire fears of easy contagion and bizarre fantasies of transmission by nonvenereal means in public places. The removal of doorknobs and the installation of swinging doors on US Navy ships and the disappearance of the metal drinking cups affixed to public water fountains in the United States in the first decades of the century were early consequences of the 'discovery' of syphilis's 'innocently transmitted infection'; and the warning to generations of middle-class children always to interpose paper between bare bottom and the public toilet seat is another trace of the horror stories about the germs of syphilis being passed to the innocent by the dirty that were rife once and are still widely believed. Every feared epidemic disease, but especially those associated with sexual license, generates a preoccupying distinction between the disease's putative carriers (which usually means just the poor and, in this part of the world, people with darker skins) and those defined – health professionals and other bureaucrats do the defining – as 'the general population.' AIDS has revived similar phobias and fears of contamination among *this* disease's version of 'the general population': white heterosexuals who do not inject themselves with drugs or have sexual relations with those who do. Like syphilis a disease of, or contracted from, dangerous others, AIDS is perceived as afflicting, in greater proportions than syphilis ever did, the already stigmatized. But syphilis was not identified with certain death, death that follows a protracted agony, as cancer was once imagined and AIDS is now held to be.

That AIDS is not a single illness but a syndrome, consisting of a seemingly open-ended list of contributing or 'presenting' illnesses which constitute (that is, qualify the patient as having) the disease, makes it more a product of definition or construction than even a very complex, multiform illness like cancer. Indeed, the contention that AIDS is invariably fatal depends partly on what doctors decided to define as AIDS – and keep in reserve as distinct earlier stages of the disease. And this decision rests on a notion no less primitively metaphorical than that of a 'full-blown' (or 'full-fledged') disease.* 'Full-blown' is the form in which the disease is inevitably fatal. As what is immature is destined to become mature, what buds to become full-blown (fledglings to become full-fledged) – the doctors' botanical or zoological metaphor makes development or evolution

* The standard definition distinguishes between people with the disease or syndrome 'fulfilling the criteria for the surveillance definition of AIDS' and a larger number infected with HIV and symptomatic 'who do not fulfill the empiric criteria for the full-blown disease. This constellation of signs and symptoms in the context of HIV infection has been termed the AIDS-related complex (ARC).' Then follows the obligatory percentage. 'It is estimated that approximately 25 percent of patients with ARC will develop full-blown disease within 3 years.' Harrison's *Principles of Internal Medicine*, 11th edition (1987), p. 1394.

The first major illness known by an acronym, the condition called AIDS does not have, as it were, natural borders. It is an illness whose identity is designed for purposes of investigation and with tabulation and surveillance by medical and other bureaucracies in view. Hence, the unselfconscious equating in the medical textbook of what is empirical with what pertains to surveillance, two notions deriving from quite different models of understanding. (AIDS is what fulfills that which is referred to as either the 'criteria for the surveillance definition' or the 'empiric criteria': HIV infection plus the presence of one or more diseases included on the roster drawn up by the disease's principal administrator of definition in the United States, the federal Centers for Disease Control in Atlanta.) This completely stipulative definition with its metaphor of maturing disease decisively influences how the illness is understood.

into AIDS the norm, the rule. I am not saying that the metaphor creates the clinical conception, but I am arguing that it does much more than just ratify it. It lends support to an interpretation of the clinical evidence which is far from proved or, yet, provable. It is simply too early to conclude, of a disease identified only seven years ago, that infection will always produce something to die from, or even that everybody who has what is defined as AIDS will die of it. (As some medical writers have speculated, the appalling mortality rates could be registering the early, mostly rapid deaths of those most vulnerable to the virus – because of diminished immune competence, because of genetic predisposition, among other possible co-factors – not the ravages of a uniformly fatal infection.) Construing the disease as divided into distinct stages was the necessary way of implementing the metaphor of 'full-blown disease.' But it also slightly weakened the notion of inevitability suggested by the metaphor. Those sensibly interested in hedging their bets about how uniformly lethal infection would prove could use the standard three-tier classification – HIV infection, AIDS-related complex (ARC), and AIDS – to entertain either of two possibilities or both: the less catastrophic one, that *not* everybody infected would 'advance' or 'graduate' from HIV infection, and the more catastrophic one, that everybody would.

It is the more catastrophic reading of the evidence that for some time has dominated debate about the disease, which means that a change in nomenclature is under way. Influential administrators of the way the disease is understood have decided that there should be no more of the false reassurance that might be had from the use of different acronyms for different stages of the disease. (It could never have been more than minimally reassuring.) Recent proposals for re-doing terminology – for instance, to phase out the category of ARC – do not challenge the construction of the disease in stages, but do place additional stress on the *continuity* of the disease process. 'Full-blown disease' is viewed as more inevitable now, and that strengthens the fatalism already in place.*

From the beginning the construction of the illness had depended on notions that separated one group of people from another – the sick from the well, people with

* The 1988 Presidential Commission on the epidemic recommended 'de-emphasizing' the use of the term ARC because it 'tends to obscure the life-threatening aspects of this stage of illness.' There is some pressure to drop the term AIDS, too. The report by the Presidential Commission pointedly used the acronym HIV for the epidemic itself, as part of a recommended shift from 'monitoring disease' to 'monitoring infection.' Again, one of the reasons given is that the present terminology masks the true gravity of the menace. ('This longstanding concentration on the clinical manifestations of AIDS rather than on all stages of HIV infection [i.e., from initial infection to seroconversion, to an antibody-positive asymptomatic stage, to full-blown AIDS] has had the unintended effect of misleading the public as to the extent of infection in the population ...') It does seem likely that the disease will, eventually, be renamed. *This* change in nomenclature would justify officially the policy of including the infected but asymptomatic among the ill.)

ARC from people with AIDS, them and us – while implying the imminent dissolution of these distinctions. However hedged, the predictions always sounded fatalistic. Thus, the frequent pronouncements by AIDS specialists and public health officials on the chances of those infected with the virus coming down with 'full-blown' disease have seemed mostly an exercise in the management of public opinion, dosing out the harrowing news in several steps. Estimates of the percentage expected to show symptoms classifying them as having AIDS within five years, which may be too low – at the time of this writing, the figure is 30 to 35 percent – are invariably followed by the assertion that 'most,' after which comes 'probably all,' those infected will eventually become ill. The critical number, then, is not the percentage of people likely to develop AIDS within a relatively short time but the *maximum* interval that could elapse between infection with HIV (described as lifelong and irreversible) and appearance of the first symptoms. As the years add up in which the illness has been tracked, so does the possible number of years between infection and becoming ill, now estimated, seven years into the epidemic, at between ten and fifteen years. This figure, which will presumably continue to be revised upward, does much to maintain the definition of AIDS as an inexorable, invariably fatal disease.

The obvious consequence of believing that all those who 'harbor' the virus will eventually come down with the illness is that those who test positive for it are regarded as people-with-AIDS, who just don't have it . . . yet. It is only a matter of time, like any death sentence. Less obviously, such people are often regarded as if they *do* have it. Testing positive for HIV (which usually means having been tested for the presence not of the virus but of antibodies to the virus) is increasingly equated with being ill. Infected *means* ill, from that point forward. 'Infected but not ill,' that invaluable notion of clinical medicine (the body 'harbors' many infections), is being superseded by biomedical concepts which, whatever their scientific justification, amount to reviving the antiscientific logic of defilement, and make infected-but-healthy a contradiction in terms. Being ill in this new sense can have many practical consequences. People are losing their jobs when it is learned that they are HIV-positive (though it is not legal in the United States to fire someone for that reason) and the temptation to conceal a positive finding must be immense. The consequences of testing HIV-positive are even more punitive for those selected populations – there will be more – upon which the government has already made testing mandatory. The US Department of Defense has announced that military personnel discovered to be HIV-positive are being removed 'from sensitive, stressful jobs,' because of evidence indicating that mere infection with the virus, in the absence of any other symptoms, produces subtle changes in mental abilities in a significant minority of virus carriers. (The evidence cited: lower scores on certain neurological tests given to some who had tested positive, which could reflect mental impairment caused by exposure to the virus, though most doctors think this extremely improbable, or could be caused – as officially acknowledged under questioning – by 'the anger, depression, fear, and panic' of people who have just learned that they are HIV-positive.) And, of course, testing positive now makes one ineligible to immigrate everywhere.

In every previous epidemic of an infectious nature, the epidemic is equivalent to the number of tabulated cases. This epidemic is regarded as consisting *now* of that figure plus a calculation about a much larger number of people apparently in good health (seemingly healthy, but doomed) who are infected. The calculations are being made and remade all the time, and pressure is building to identify these people, and to tag them. With the most up-to-date biomedical testing, it is possible to create a new class of lifetime pariahs, the future ill. But the result of this radical expansion of the notion of illness created by the triumph of modern medical scrutiny also seems a throwback to the past, before the era of medical triumphalism, when illnesses were innumerable, mysterious, and the progression from being seriously ill to dying was something normal (not, as now, medicine's lapse or failure, destined to be corrected). AIDS, in which people are understood as ill before they are ill; which produces a seemingly innumerable array of symptom-illnesses; for which there are only palliatives; and which brings to many a social death that precedes the physical one – AIDS reinstates something like a premodern experience of illness, as described in Donne's

Devotions, in which 'every thing that disorders a faculty and the function of that is a sicknesse,' which starts when we

> are preafflicted, super-afflicted with these jelousies and sus-
> pitions, and apprehensions of Sicknes, before we can cal it a
> sicknes; we are not sure we are ill; one hand askes the other
> by the pulse, and our eye asks our own urine, how we
> do ... we are tormented with sicknes, and cannot stay till
> the torment come ...

whose agonizing outreach to every part of the body makes a real cure chimerical, since what 'is but an acci-dent, but a symptom of the main disease, is so violent, that the Phisician must attend the cure of that' rather than 'the cure of the disease it self,' and whose con-sequence is abandonment:

> As Sicknesse is the greatest misery, so the greatest misery
> of sicknes is solitude; when the infectiousnes of the disease
> deterrs them who should assist, from comming; even the
> Phisician dares scarse come ... it is an Outlawry, an Ex-
> communication upon the patient ...

In premodern medicine, illness is described as it is experienced intuitively, as a relation of outside and inside: an interior sensation or something to be discerned on the body's surface, by sight (or just below, by listen-ing, palpating), which is confirmed when the interior is opened to viewing (in surgery, in autopsy). Modern – that is, effective – medicine is characterized by far more complex notions of what is to be observed inside the body: not just the disease's results (damaged organs) but its cause (microorganisms), and by a far more intricate typology of illness.

In the older era of artisanal diagnoses, being examined produced an immediate verdict, immediate as the physician's willingness to speak. Now an examination means tests. And being tested introduces a time lapse that, given the unavoidably industrial character of competent medical testing, can stretch out for weeks: an agonizing delay for those who think they are awaiting a death sentence or an acquittal. Many are reluctant to be tested out of dread of the verdict, out of fear of being put on a list that could bring future discrimination or worse, and out of fatalism (what good would it do?). The usefulness of self-examination for the early detection of certain common cancers, much less likely to be fatal if treated before they are very advanced, is now widely understood. Early detection of an illness thought to be inexorable and incurable cannot seem to bring any advantage.

Like other diseases that arouse feelings of shame, AIDS is often a secret, but not from the patient. A cancer diagnosis was frequently concealed from patients by their families; an AIDS diagnosis is at least as often concealed from their families by patients. And as with other grave illnesses regarded as more than just illnesses, many people with AIDS are drawn to whole-body rather than illness-specific treatments, which are thought to be either ineffectual or too dangerous. (The disparagement of effective, scientific medicine for offering treatments that are *merely* illness-specific, and likely to be toxic, is a recurrent misconjecture of opinion that regards itself as enlightened.) This disastrous choice is still being made by some people with cancer, an illness that surgery and drugs can often cure. And a predictable mix of superstition and resignation is leading some people with AIDS to refuse antiviral chemotherapy, which, even in the absence of a cure, has proved of some effectiveness (in slowing down the syndrome's progress and in staving off some common presenting illnesses), and instead to seek to heal themselves, often under the auspices of some 'alternative medicine' guru. But subjecting an emaciated body to the purification of a macrobiotic diet is about as helpful in treating AIDS as having oneself bled, the 'holistic' medical treatment of choice in the era of Donne.

Chapter Four

Etymologically, patient means sufferer. It is not suffering as such that is most deeply feared but suffering that degrades.

That illness can be not only an epic of suffering but the occasion of some kind of self-transcendence is affirmed by sentimental literature and, more convincingly, by case histories offered by doctor-writers. Some illnesses seem more apt than others for this kind of meditation. Oliver Sacks uses catastrophic neurological illness as the material for his portraits of suffering and self-transcendence, diminishment and exaltation. His great forerunner, Sir Thomas Browne, used tuberculosis for a similar purpose, to ruminate about illness in general, in 'A Letter to a Friend, Upon Occasion of the Death of his Intimate Friend' (1657), making pre-Romantic sense out of some of the familiar stereotypes about tuberculosis: that it is a distinctive manner of being ill ('this being a lingring Disease') and a distinctive manner of dying ('his soft Death'). A fiction about soft or easy deaths – in fact, dying of tuberculosis was often hard and extremely painful – is part of the mythology of most diseases that are not considered shameful or demeaning.

In contrast to the soft death imputed to tuberculosis, AIDS, like cancer, leads to a hard death. The metaphorized illnesses that haunt the collective imagination are all hard deaths, or envisaged as such. Being deadly is not in itself enough to produce terror. It is not even necessary, as in the puzzling case of leprosy, perhaps the most stigmatized of all diseases, although rarely fatal and extremely difficult to transmit. Cancer is more feared than heart disease, although someone who has had a coronary is more likely to die of heart disease in the next few years than someone who has cancer is likely to die of cancer. A heart attack is an event but it does not give someone a new identity, turning the patient into one of 'them.' It is not transforming except in the sense of a transformation into something better: inspired by fear, the cardiac patient acquires good habits of exercise and diet, starts to lead a more prudent, healthier life. And it is often thought to produce, if only because it can be instantaneous, an easy death.

The most terrifying illnesses are those perceived not just as lethal but as dehumanizing, literally so. What was expressed in the rabies phobia of nineteenth-century France, with its countless pseudo-cases of contamination by animals newly turned 'bestial' and even of 'spontaneous' rabies (actual cases of rabies, *la rage*, were extremely rare), was the fantasy that infection transformed people into maddened animals – unleashing uncontrollable sexual, blasphemous impulses – not the fact that it was indeed, until Pasteur's discovery of a treatment in 1885, invariably fatal. And while cholera killed fewer people in Western Europe in the nineteenth century than smallpox did, it was more feared, because of the suddenness with which it struck and the indignity of the symptoms: fulminant diarrhea and vomiting, whose result anticipated the horror of post-mortem decomposition. Within several hours radical dehydration shrank the patient into a wizened caricature of his or her former self, the skin turned bluish-black (overwhelming, transfixing fear is still, in French, *une peur bleue*), the body became cold; death followed the same day or soon after.

Polio's effects could be horrifying – it withered the body – but it did not mark or rot the flesh: it was not repulsive. Further, polio affected the body only, though that may seem ruin enough, not the face. The relatively appropriate, unmetaphorical reaction to polio owes much to the privileged status of the face, so determining of our evaluation of physical beauty and of physical ruin. All the debunking of the Cartesian separation of *mind* and body by modern philosophy and modern science has not reduced by one iota this culture's conviction of the separation of *face* and body, which influences every aspect of manners, fashion, sexual appreciation, aesthetic sensibility – virtually all our notions of appropriateness. This separation is a main point of one of

European culture's principal iconographical traditions, the depiction of Christian martyrdom, with its astounding schism between what is inscribed on the face and what is happening to the body. Those innumerable images of Saint Sebastian, Saint Agatha, Saint Lawrence (but not of Christ himself), with the face demonstrating its effortless superiority to the atrocious things that are being inflicted down there. Below, the ruin of the body. Above, a person, incarnated in the face, who looks away, usually up, not registering pain or fear; already elsewhere. (Only Christ, both Son of Man and Son of God, suffers in his face: has his Passion.) Our very notion of the person, of dignity, depends on the separation of face from body,* on the possibility that the face may be exempt, or exempt itself, from what is happening to the body. And however lethal, illnesses like heart attacks and influenza that do not damage or deform the face never arouse the deepest dread.

Not every kind of alteration to the face is perceived as repulsive or shaming. The most dreaded are those that

---

* There can be no real argument against the aristocracy of the face, only definitive raillery. An obsession with the pretentiousness of the division between face and body is central in Gombrowicz's *Ferdydurke*, which keeps reproposing that the body is parts, each with an independent life, and the face is just another body part. The point of view from which Gombrowicz launches his post-Rabelaisian satire on eros and on social class is that of an enforced, humiliating return to childhood – not of the enforced humiliations of illness. That is, Gombrowicz's novel is a comedy, not a tragedy.

seem like mutations into animality (the leper's 'lion face') or a kind of rot (as in syphilis). Underlying some of the moral judgments attached to disease are aesthetic judgments about the beautiful and the ugly, the clean and the unclean, the familiar and the alien or uncanny. (More accurately, these are judgments that originate before the stage at which aesthetic and moral categories split apart and, eventually, come to seem opposed.) What counts more than the amount of disfigurement is that it reflects underlying, ongoing changes, the dissolution of the person. Smallpox also disfigures, pitting the face; but the marks of smallpox don't get worse. Indeed, they are precisely the stigmata of a survivor. The marks on the face of a leper, a syphilitic, someone with AIDS are the signs of a progressive mutation, decomposition; something organic.

Sinister characterizations of the organic proliferated in the nineteenth century to describe both the disease and its cause. Specific diseases, such as cholera, as well as the state of being generally prone to illness, were thought to be caused by an 'infected' (or 'foul') atmosphere, effusions spontaneously generated from something unclean. Usually identified (first by its bad smell) as decaying organic matter, this disease-carrying atmosphere came to be identified with urban rather than rural squalor, and with garbage, rot, the proximity of cemeteries. These claims were eventually defeated by the discoveries by Pasteur and Koch of the role played by specific microorganisms. By 1880 the scientific community no longer believed in miasma, as these effusions were called, or in spontaneous generation. (In 1883, a year after Koch discovered the tubercle bacillus, he discovered the water-borne bacillus that causes cholera.) But even after the defeat of the miasmic theory by the germ theory of contagion, miasma lived on, shorn of its first-order causative status, as a kind of vague co-factor in the explanation of many illnesses. The conviction that living in dark, dirty cities causes (or at least produces a susceptibility to) tuberculosis is a version of the miasma theory, and continued to be given credence well into this century, long after the actual cause of tuberculosis had been discovered. It seems that something like what is supplied by miasma, the generalizing of infection into an atmosphere, is required to moralize a disease.

In the wake of its rejection by scientists, the theory inspired at least one great work of art: the opera Debussy made from Maeterlinck's play *Pelléas et Mélisande*, a sort of *Tristan und Isolde* relocated in the world of miasma. It is right that *Pelléas et Mélisande*, in which everyone avows feelings of weakness and being lost, and some are already ailing; with its old, decaying castle that lets in no light; where the ground is full of subterranean terrors and dank or watery depths into which one can fall – all the correlatives of miasma, minus the stench – seems, to us, supremely a portrait of *psychological* sickness, of neurosis. For precisely as the category of generic sickliness was phased out of nineteenth-century medical thinking by the new understanding of the extreme specificity of what causes illness, it migrated to the expanding domain of psychology. The physically sickly person became the neurasthenic or neurotic person. And the idea of an organically contaminated, objectively pathogenic environment reappeared in the notion of a psychologically contaminated ambiance that produced a disposition to mental illness.

The notion did not remain confined to the domain of psychology and, with psychology's new credibility as science, returned to reinfluence medicine. The widely held view that many or even most diseases are not 'really' physical but mental (more conservatively, 'psychosomatic') perpetuates the form of the miasmic theory – with its surplus of causality, surplus of meaning – in a new version that has been extremely successful in the twentieth century. The theory that psychological miasma (depression, funk) can cause physical illness has been tried out with varying degrees of respectability on many diseases, including cancer. And one way in which AIDS, some of whose metaphors overlap those of cancer, seems very different from cancer, that illness saturated with distinctively modern evaluations of energy and of disaster, and is experienced as a throwback to premodern diseases like leprosy and syphilis, is that no one is tempted, not yet at least, to psychologize it.

Chapter Five

'Plague' is the principal metaphor by which the AIDS epidemic is understood. And because of AIDS, the popular misidentification of cancer as an epidemic, even a plague, seems to be receding: AIDS has banalized cancer.

Plague, from the Latin *plaga* (stroke, wound), has long been used metaphorically as the highest standard of collective calamity, evil, scourge – Procopius, in his masterpiece of calumny, *The Secret History*, called the Emperor Justinian worse than the plague ('fewer escaped') – as well as being a general name for many frightening diseases. Although the disease to which the word is permanently affixed produced the most lethal of recorded epidemics, being experienced as a pitiless slayer is not necessary for a disease to be regarded as plague-like. Leprosy, very rarely fatal now, was not much more so when at its greatest epidemic strength, between about 1050 and 1350. And syphilis has been regarded as a plague – Blake speaks of 'the youthful Harlot's curse' that 'blights with plagues the Marriage hearse' – not because it killed often, but because it was disgracing, disempowering, disgusting.

It is usually epidemics that are thought of as plagues. And these mass incidences of illness are understood as inflicted, not just endured. Considering illness as a punishment is the oldest idea of what causes illness, and an idea opposed by all attention to the ill that deserves the noble name of medicine. Hippocrates, who wrote several treatises on epidemics, specifically ruled out 'the wrath of God' as a cause of bubonic plague. But the illnesses interpreted in antiquity as punishments, like the plague in *Oedipus*, were not thought to be shameful, as leprosy and subsequently syphilis were to be. Diseases, insofar as they acquired meaning, were collective calamities, and judgments on a community. Only injuries and disabilities, not diseases, were thought of as individually merited. For an analogy in the literature of antiquity to the modern sense of a shaming, isolating disease, one would have to turn to Philoctetes and his stinking wound.

The most feared diseases, those that are not simply fatal but transform the body into something alienating like leprosy and syphilis and cholera and (in the imagination of many) cancer, are the ones that seem particularly susceptible to promotion to 'plague.' Leprosy and syphilis were the first illnesses to be consistently described as repulsive. It was syphilis, that, in the earliest descriptions by doctors at the end of the fifteenth century, generated a version of the metaphors that flourish around AIDS: of a disease that was not only repulsive and retributive but collectively invasive. Although Erasmus, the most influential European pedagogue of the early sixteenth century, described syphilis as 'nothing but a kind of leprosy' (by 1529 he called it 'something worse than leprosy'), it had already been understood as something different, because sexually transmitted. Paracelsus speaks (in Donne's paraphrase) of 'that foule contagious disease which then had invaded mankind in a few places, and since overflowes in all, that for punishment of generall licentiousnes God first inflicted that disease.' Thinking of syphilis as a punishment for an individual's transgression was for a long time, virtually until the disease became easily curable, not really distinct from regarding it as retribution for the licentiousness of a community – as with AIDS now, in the rich industrial countries. In contrast to cancer, understood in a modern way as a disease incurred by (and revealing of) individuals, AIDS is understood in a premodern way, as a disease incurred by people both as individuals and as members of a 'risk group' – that neutral-sounding, bureaucratic, category which also revives the archaic idea of a tainted community that illness has judged.

Not every account of plague or plague-like diseases, of course, is a vehicle for lurid stereotypes about illness and the ill. The effort to think critically, historically, about illness (about disaster generally) was attempted throughout the eighteenth century; say, from Defoe's *A*

Journal of the Plague Year (1722) to Alessandro Manzoni's *The Betrothed* (1827). Defoe's historical fiction, purporting to be an eyewitness account of bubonic plague in London in 1665, does not further any understanding of the plague as punishment or, a later part of the script, as a transforming experience. And Manzoni, in his lengthy account of the passage of plague through the duchy of Milan in 1630, is avowedly committed to presenting a more accurate, less reductive view than his historical sources. But even these two complex narratives reinforce some of the perennial, simplifying ideas about plague.

One feature of the usual script for plague: the disease invariably comes from somewhere else. The names for syphilis, when it began its epidemic sweep through Europe in the last decade of the fifteenth century, are an exemplary illustration of the need to make a dreaded disease foreign.* It was the 'French pox' to the English, *morbus Germanicus* to the Parisians, the Naples sickness to the Florentines, the Chinese disease to the Japanese. But

---

* As noted in the first accounts of the disease: 'This malady received from different peoples whom it affected different names,' writes Giovanni di Vigo in 1514. Like earlier treatises on syphilis, written in Latin – by Nicolo Leoniceno (1497) and by Juan Almenar (1502) – the one by di Vigo calls it *morbus Gallicus*, the French disease. (Excerpts from this and other accounts of the period, including *Syphilis; Or a Poetical History of the French Disease* [1530] by Girolamo Fracastoro, who coined the name that prevailed, are in *Classic Descriptions of Disease*, edited by Ralph H. Major [1932].) Moralistic explanations abounded from the beginning. In 1495, a year after the epidemic started, the Emperor Maximilian issued an edict declaring syphilis to be an affliction from God for the sins of men.

what may seem like a joke about the inevitability of chauvinism reveals a more important truth: that there is a link between imagining disease and imagining foreignness. It lies perhaps in the very concept of wrong, which is archaically identical with the non-us, the alien. A polluting person is always wrong, as Mary Douglas has observed. The inverse is also true: a person judged to be wrong is regarded as, at least potentially, a source of pollution.

The foreign place of origin of important illnesses, as of drastic changes in the weather, may be no more remote than a neighboring country. Illness is a species of invasion, and indeed is often carried by soldiers. Manzoni's account of the plague of 1630 (chapters 31 to 37) begins:

> The plague which the Tribunal of Health had feared might enter the Milanese provinces with the German troops had in fact entered, as is well known; and it is also well known that it did not stop there, but went on to invade and depopulate a large part of Italy.

Defoe's chronicle of the plague of 1665 begins similarly,

The theory that syphilis came from even farther than a neighboring country, that it was an entirely new disease in Europe, a disease of the New World brought back to the Old by sailors of Columbus who had contracted it in America, became the accepted explanation of the origin of syphilis in the sixteenth century and is still widely credited. It is worth noting that the earliest medical writers on syphilis did not accept the dubious theory. Leoniceno's *Libellus de Epidemia, quam vulgo morbum Gallicum vocant* starts by taking up the question of whether 'the French disease under another name was common to the ancients,' and says he believes firmly that it was.

with a flurry of ostentatiously scrupulous speculation about its foreign origin:

> It was about the beginning of September, 1664, that I, among the rest of my neighbours, heard in ordinary discourse that the plague was returned again in Holland; for it had been very violent there, and particularly at Amsterdam and Rotterdam, in the year 1663, whither, they say, it was brought, some said from Italy, others from the Levant, among some goods which were brought home by their Turkey fleet; others said it was brought from Candia; others from Cyprus. It mattered not from whence it came; but all agreed it was come into Holland again.

The bubonic plague that reappeared in London in the 1720s had arrived from Marseilles, which was where plague in the eighteenth century was usually thought to enter Western Europe: brought by seamen, then transported by soldiers and merchants. By the nineteenth century the foreign origin was usually more exotic, the means of transport less specifically imagined, and the illness itself had become phantasmagorical, symbolic.

At the end of *Crime and Punishment* Raskolnikov dreams of plague: 'He dreamt that the whole world was condemned to a terrible new strange plague that had come to Europe from the depths of Asia.' At the beginning of the sentence it is 'the whole world,' which turns out by the end of the sentence to be 'Europe,' afflicted by a lethal visitation from Asia. Dostoevsky's model is undoubtedly cholera, called Asiatic cholera, long endemic in Bengal, which had rapidly become and remained through most of the nineteenth century a worldwide epidemic disease. Part of the centuries-old conception of Europe as a privileged cultural entity is that it is a place which is colonized by lethal diseases coming from elsewhere. Europe is assumed to be by rights free of disease. (And Europeans have been astoundingly callous about the far more devastating extent to which they – as invaders, as colonists – have introduced *their* lethal diseases to the exotic, 'primitive' world: think of the ravages of smallpox, influenza, and cholera on the aboriginal populations of the Americas and Australia.) The tenacity of the connection of exotic origin with dreaded disease is one reason why cholera, of which there were four great outbreaks in Europe in the nineteenth century, each with a lower death toll than the preceding one, has continued to be more memorable than smallpox, whose ravages increased as the century went on (half a million died in the European smallpox pandemic of the early 1870s) but which could not be construed as, plague-like, a disease with a non-European origin.

Plagues are no longer 'sent', as in Biblical and Greek antiquity, for the question of agency has blurred. Instead, peoples are 'visited' by plagues. And the visitations recur, as is taken for granted in the subtitle of Defoe's narrative, which explains, that it is about that 'which happened in London during the Last Great Visitation in 1665.' Even for non-Europeans, lethal disease may be called a visitation. But a visitation on 'them' is invariably described as different from one on 'us.' 'I believe that about one half of the whole people was carried off by this visitation,' wrote the English traveler Alexander Kinglake, reaching Cairo at a time of the bubonic plague (sometimes called 'oriental plague'). 'The Orientals, however, have more quiet fortitude than Europeans under afflictions of this sort.' Kinglake's influential book *Eothen* (1844) – suggestively subtitled 'Traces of Travel Brought Home from the East' – illustrates many of the enduring Eurocentric presumptions about others, starting from the fantasy that peoples with little reason to expect exemption from misfortune have a lessened capacity to *feel* misfortune. Thus it is believed that Asians (or the poor, or blacks, or Africans, or Muslims) don't suffer or don't grieve as Europeans (or whites) do. The fact that illness is associated with the poor – who are, from the perspective of the privileged, aliens in one's midst – reinforces the association of illness with the foreign: with an exotic, often primitive place.

Thus, illustrating the classic script for plague, AIDS is thought to have started in the 'dark continent,' then spread to Haiti, then to the United States and to Europe, then ... It is understood as a tropical disease: another infestation from the so-called Third World, which is after all where most people in the world live, as well as a scourge of the *tristes tropiques*. Africans who detect racist stereotypes in much of the speculation about the geographical origin of AIDS are not wrong. (Nor are they wrong in thinking that depictions of Africa as the cradle of AIDS must feed anti-African prejudices in Europe and Asia.) The subliminal connection made to notions about a primitive past and the many hypotheses that have been fielded about possible transmission from animals (a disease of green monkeys? African swine fever?) cannot help but activate a familiar set of stereotypes about animality, sexual license, and blacks. In Zaire and other countries in Central Africa where AIDS is killing tens of thousands, the counterreaction has begun. Many doctors, academics, journalists, government officials, and other educated people believe that the virus was sent to Africa from the United States, an act of bacteriological warfare (whose aim was to decrease the African birth rate) which got out of hand and has returned to afflict its perpetrators. A common African version of this belief about the disease's provenance has the virus fabricated in a CIA–Army laboratory in Maryland, sent from there to Africa, and brought back to its country of origin by American homosexual missionaries returning from Africa to Maryland.*

---

* The rumor may not have originated as a KGB-sponsored 'disinformation' campaign, but it received a crucial push from Soviet propaganda specialists. In October 1985 the Soviet weekly *Literaturnaya Gazeta* published an article alleging that the AIDS virus had been engineered by the US government during biological-warfare research at Fort Detrick, Maryland, and was being spread abroad by US servicemen who had been used as guinea pigs. The source cited was an article in the Indian newspaper *Patriot*. Repeated on Moscow's 'Radio Peace and Progress' in English, the story was taken up by newspapers and magazines throughout the world. A year later it was featured on the front page of London's conservative, mass-circulation *Sunday Express*. ('The killer AIDS virus was artificially created by American scientists

At first it was assumed that AIDS must become wide-spread elsewhere in the same catastrophic form in which it has emerged in Africa, and those who still think this will eventually happen invariably invoke the Black Death. The plague metaphor is an essential vehicle of the most pessimistic reading of the epidemiological prospects. From classic fiction to the latest journalism, the standard plague story is of inexorability, inescapability. The unprepared are taken by surprise; those observing the recommended precautions are struck down as well. *All* succumb when the story is told by an omniscient narrator, as in Poe's parable 'The Masque of the Red Death' (1842), inspired by an account of a ball held in Paris during the cholera epidemic of 1832. Almost all – if the story is told from the point of view of a traumatized witness, who will be a benumbed survivor, as in Jean Giono's Stendhalian novel *Horseman on the Roof* (1951), in which a young Italian nobleman in exile wanders through cholera-stricken southern France in the 1830s.

*

during laboratory experiments which went disastrously wrong – and a massive cover-up has kept the secret from the world until today.') Though ignored by most American newspapers, the *Sunday Express* story was recycled in virtually every other country. As recently as the summer of 1987, it appeared in newspapers in Kenya, Peru, Sudan, Nigeria, Senegal, and Mexico. Gorbachev-era policies have since produced an official denial of the allegations by two eminent members of the Soviet Academy of Sciences, which was published in *Izvestia* in late October 1987. But the story is still being repeated – from Mexico to Zaire, from Australia to Greece.

Plagues are invariably regarded as judgments on society, and the metaphoric inflation of AIDS into such a judgment also accustoms people to the inevitability of global spread. This is a traditional use of sexually transmitted diseases; to be described as punishments not just of individuals but of a group ('generall licentiousnes'). Not only venereal diseases have been used in this way to identify transgressing or vicious populations. Interpreting any catastrophic epidemic as a sign of moral laxity or political decline was as common until the later part of the last century as associating dreaded diseases with foreignness. (Or with despised and feared minorities.) And the assignment of fault is not contradicted by cases that do not fit. The Methodist preachers in England who connected the cholera epidemic of 1832 with drunkenness (the temperance movement was just starting) were not understood to be claiming that *everybody* who got cholera was a drunkard; there is always room for 'innocent victims' (children, young women). Tuberculosis, in its identity as a disease of the poor (rather than of the 'sensitive'), was also linked by late-nineteenth-century reformers to alcoholism. Responses to illnesses associated with sinners and the poor invariably recommended the adoption of middle-class values: the regular habits, productivity, and emotional self-control to which drunkenness was thought the chief impediment.* Health itself was eventually identified with

* According to the more comprehensive diagnosis favoured by secular reformers, cholera was the result of poor diet and 'indulgence

140

these values, which were religious as well as mercantile, health being evidence of virtue as disease was of depravity. The dictum that cleanliness is next to godliness is to be taken quite literally. The succession of cholera epidemics in the nineteenth century shows a steady waning of religious interpretations of the disease; more precisely, these increasingly coexisted with other explanations. Although, by the time of the epidemic of 1866, cholera was commonly understood not simply as a divine punishment but as the consequence of remediable defects of sanitation, it was still regarded as the scourge of the sinful. A writer in *The New York Times* declared (April 22, 1866): 'Cholera is especially the punishment of neglect of sanitary laws; it is the curse of the dirty, the intemperate, and the degraded.'†

That it now seems unimaginable for cholera or a similar disease to be regarded in this way signifies not a lessened capacity to moralize about diseases but only a change in the kind of illnesses that are used didactically. Cholera was perhaps the last major epidemic disease fully qualifying for plague status for almost a century. (I mean cholera as a European and American, therefore a nineteenth-century, disease; until 1817 there had never

---

in irregular habits.' Officials of the Central Board of Health in London warned that there were no specific treatments for the disease, and advised paying attention to fresh air and cleanliness, though 'the true preventatives are a healthy body and a cheerful, unruffled mind.' Quoted in R. J. Morris, *Cholera 1832* (1976).

† Quoted in Charles E. Rosenberg, *The Cholera Years: The United States in 1832, 1849, and 1866* (1962).

been a cholera epidemic outside the Far East.) Influenza, which would seem more plague-like than any other epidemic in this century if loss of life were the main criterion, and which struck as suddenly as cholera and killed as quickly, usually in a few days, was never viewed metaphorically as a plague. Nor was a more recent epidemic, polio. One reason why plague notions were not invoked is that these epidemics did not have enough of the attributes perennially ascribed to plagues. (For instance, polio was construed as typically a disease of children – of the innocent.) The more important reason is that there has been a shift in the focus of the moralistic exploitation of illness. This shift, to diseases that can be interpreted as judgments on the individual, makes it harder to use epidemic disease as such. For a long time cancer was the illness that best fitted this secular culture's need to blame and punish and censor through the imagery of disease. Cancer was a disease of an individual, and understood as the result not of an action but rather of a failure to act (to be prudent, to exert proper self-control, or to be properly expressive). In the twentieth century it has become almost impossible to moralize about epidemics – except those which are transmitted sexually.

The persistence of the belief that illness reveals, and is a punishment for, moral laxity or turpitude can be seen in another way, by noting the persistence of descriptions of disorder or corruption as a disease. So indispensable has been the plague metaphor in bringing summary judgments about social crisis that its use hardly abated during the era when collective diseases were no longer treated so moralistically – the time between the influenza and encephalitis pandemics of the early and mid 1920s and the acknowledgment of a new, mysterious epidemic illness in the early 1980s – and when great infectious epidemics were so often and confidently proclaimed a thing of the past.* The plague metaphor was common in the 1930s as a synonym for social and psychic catastrophe. Evocations of plague of this type usually go with rant, with antiliberal attitudes: think of Artaud on theatre and plague, of Wilhelm Reich on 'emotional plague.' And such a generic 'diagnosis' necessarily promotes antihistorical thinking. A theodicy as well as a demonology, it not only stipulates something emblematic of evil but makes this the bearer of a rough, terrible justice. In Karel Čapek's *The White Plague* (1937), the loathsome pestilence that has appeared in a state where fascism has come to power afflicts only those over the age of forty, those who could be held morally responsible.

Written on the eve of the Nazi takeover of Czechoslovakia, Čapek's allegorical play is something of an anomaly – the use of the plague metaphor to convey the

---

* As recently as 1983, the historian William H. McNeill, author of *Plagues and Peoples*, started his review of a new history of the Black Death by asserting: 'One of the things that separate us from our ancestors and make contemporary experience profoundly different from that of other ages is the disappearance of epidemic disease as a serious factor in human life' (*The New York Review of Books*, July 21, 1983). The Eurocentric presumption of this and many similar statements hardly needs pointing out.

menace of what is defined as barbaric by a mainstream European liberal. The play's mysterious, grisly malady is something like leprosy, a rapid, invariably fatal leprosy that is supposed to have come, of course, from Asia. But Čapek is not interested in identifying political evil with the incursion of the foreign. He scores his didactic points by focusing not on the disease itself but on the management of information about it by scientists, journalists, and politicians. The most famous specialist in the disease harangues a reporter ('The disease of the hour, you might say. A good five million have died of it to date, twenty million have it and at least three times as many are going about their business, blithely unaware of the marble-like, marble-sized spots on their bodies'); chides a fellow doctor for using the popular terms, 'the white plague' and 'Peking leprosy,' instead of the scientific name, 'the Cheng Syndrome'; fantasizes about how his clinic's work on identifying the new virus and finding a cure ('every clinic in the world has an intensive research program') will add to the prestige of science and win a Nobel Prize for its discoverer; revels in hyperbole when it is thought a cure has been found ('it was the most dangerous disease in all history, worse than the bubonic plague'); and outlines plans for sending those with symptoms to well-guarded detention camps ('Given that every carrier of the disease is a potential spreader of the disease, we *must* protect the uncontaminated from the contaminated. All sentimentality in this regard is fatal and therefore criminal'.) However cartoonish Čapek's ironies may seem, they are a not improbable sketch of catastrophe (medical, ecological) as a managed public event in modern mass society. And however conventionally he deploys the plague metaphor, as an agency of retribution (in the end the plague strikes down the dictator himself), Čapek's feel for public relations leads him to make explicit in the play the understanding of disease *as* a metaphor. The eminent doctor declares the accomplishments of science to be as nothing compared with the merits of the dictator, about to launch a war, 'who has averted a far worse scourge: the scourge of anarchy, the leprosy of corruption, the epidemic of barbaric liberty, the plague of social disintegration fatally sapping the organism of our nation.'

Camus's *The Plague*, which appeared a decade later, is a far less literal use of plague by another great European liberal, as subtle as Čapek's *The White Plague* is schematic. Camus's novel is not, as is sometimes said, a political allegory in which the outbreak of bubonic plague in a Mediterranean port city represents the Nazi occupation. This plague is not retributive. Camus is not protesting anything, not corruption or tyranny, not even mortality. The plague is no more or less than an exemplary event, the irruption of death that gives life its seriousness. His use of plague, more epitome than metaphor, is detached, stoic, aware – it is not about bringing judgment. But, as in Čapek's play, characters in Camus's novel declare how unthinkable it is to have a plague in the twentieth century . . . as if the belief that such a calamity could not happen, could not happen *anymore*, means that it must.

Chapter Six

The emergence of a new catastrophic epidemic, when for several decades it had been confidently assumed that such calamities belonged to the past, would not be enough to revive the moralistic inflation of an epidemic into a 'plague.' It was necessary that the epidemic be one whose most common means of transmission is sexual.

Cotton Mather called syphilis a punishment 'which the Just Judgment of God has reserved for our Late Ages.' Recalling this and other nonsense uttered about syphilis from the end of the fifteenth to the early twentieth centuries, one should hardly be surprised that many want to view AIDS metaphorically – as, plague-like, a moral judgment on society. Professional fulminators can't resist the rhetorical opportunity offered by a sexually transmitted disease that is lethal. Thus, the fact that AIDS is predominantly a heterosexually transmitted illness in the countries where it first emerged in epidemic form has not prevented such guardians of public morals as Jesse Helms and Norman Podhoretz from depicting it as a visitation specially aimed at (and deservedly incurred by) Western homosexuals, while another Reagan-era celebrity, Pat Buchanan, orates about 'AIDS and Moral Bankruptcy,' and Jerry Falwell offers the generic diagnosis that 'AIDS is God's judgment on a society that does not live by His rules.' What is surprising is not that the AIDS epidemic has been exploited in this way but that such cant has been confined to so predictable a sector of bigots; the official discourse about AIDS invariably includes admonitions against bigotry.

The pronouncements of those who claim to speak for God can mostly be discounted as the rhetoric regularly prompted by sexually transmitted illness – from Cotton Mather's judgment to recent statements by two leading Brazilian clerics, Bishop Falcão of Brasilia, who declares AIDS to be 'the consequence of moral decadence,' and the Cardinal of Rio de Janeiro, Eugenio Sales, who wants it both ways, describing AIDS as 'God's punishment' and as 'the revenge of nature.' More interesting, because their purposes are more complex, are the secular sponsors of this sort of invective. Authoritarian political ideologies have a vested interest in promoting fear, a sense of the imminence of takeover by aliens – and real diseases are useful material. Epidemic diseases usually elicit a call to ban the entry of foreigners, immigrants. And xenophobic propaganda has always depicted immigrants as bearers of disease (in the late nineteenth century: cholera, yellow fever, typhoid fever, tuberculosis). It seems logical that the political figure in France who represents the most extreme nativist, racist views, Jean-Marie Le Pen, has attempted a strategy of fomenting fear of this new alien peril, insisting that AIDS is not just infectious but contagious, and calling for mandatory nationwide testing and the quarantine of everyone carrying the virus. And AIDS is a gift to the present regime in South Africa, whose Foreign Minister declared recently, evoking the incidence of the illness among the mine workers imported from neighboring all-black countries: 'The terrorists are now coming to us with a weapon more terrible than Marxism: AIDS.'

The AIDS epidemic serves as an ideal projection for First World political paranoia. Not only is the so-called AIDS virus the quintessential invader from the Third World. It can stand for any mythological menace. In this country, AIDS has so far evoked less pointedly racist reactions than in Europe, including the Soviet Union, where the African origin of the disease is stressed. Here it is as much a reminder of feelings associated with the menace of the Second World as it is an image of being overrun by the Third. Predictably, the public voices in this country most committed to drawing moral lessons from the AIDS epidemic, such as Norman Podhoretz, are those whose main theme is worry about America's will to maintain its bellicosity, its expenditures on armaments, its firm anti-communist stance, and who find everywhere evidence of the decline of American political and imperial authority. Denunciations of 'the gay plague' are part of a much larger complaint, common among antiliberals in the West and many exiles from the Russian bloc, about contemporary permissiveness of all kinds: a now-familiar diatribe against the 'soft' West, with its hedonism, its vulgar sexy music, its indulgence in drugs, its disabled family life, which have sapped the will to stand up to communism. AIDS is a favorite concern of those who translate their political agenda into questions of group psychology: of national self-esteem and self-confidence. Although these specialists in ugly feelings insist that AIDS is a punishment for deviant sex, what moves them is not just, or even principally, homophobia. Even more important is the utility of AIDS in pursuing one of the main activities of the so-called neo-conservatives, the Kulturkampf against all that is called, for short (and inaccurately), the 1960s. A whole politics of 'the will' – of intolerance, of paranoia, of fear of political weakness – has fastened on this disease.

AIDS is such an apt goad to familiar consensus-building fears that have been cultivated for several generations, like fear of 'subversion' – and to fears that have surfaced more recently, of uncontrollable pollution and of unstoppable migration from the Third World – that it would seem inevitable that AIDS be envisaged in this society as something total, civilization-threatening. And raising the disease's metaphorical stature by keeping alive fears of its easy transmissibility, its imminent spread, does not diminish its status as, mainly, a consequence of illicit acts (or of economic and cultural backwardness). That it is a punishment for deviant behavior and that it threatens the innocent – these two notions about AIDS

149

are hardly in contradiction. Such is the extraordinary potency and efficacy of the plague metaphor: it allows a disease to be regarded both as something incurred by vulnerable 'others' and as (potentially) everyone's disease.

Still, it is one thing to emphasize how the disease menaces everybody (in order to incite fear and confirm prejudice), quite another to argue (in order to defuse prejudice and reduce stigma) that eventually AIDS will, directly or indirectly, affect everybody. Recently these same mythologists who have been eager to use AIDS for ideological mobilization against deviance have backed away from the most panic-inspiring estimates of the illness. They are among the most vocal of those who insist that infection will *not* spread to 'the general population' and have turned their attention to denouncing 'hysteria' or 'frenzy' about AIDS. Behind what they now consider the excessive publicity given the disease, they discern the desire to placate an all-powerful minority by agreeing to regard 'their' disease as 'ours' – further evidence of the sway of nefarious 'liberal' values and of America's spiritual decline. Making AIDS everyone's problem and therefore a subject on which everyone needs to be educated, charge the antiliberal AIDS mythologists, subverts our understanding of the difference between 'us' and 'them'; indeed, exculpates or at least makes irrelevant moral judgments about 'them.' (In such rhetoric the disease continues to be identified almost exclusively with homosexuality, and specifically the practice of sodomy.) 'Has America become a country where classroom discussion of the Ten Commandments is impermissible but teacher instructions in safe sodomy are to be mandatory?' inquires Pat Buchanan, protesting the 'foolish' proposal made in the report of the recent Presidential Commission on the epidemic, chaired by Admiral Watkins, to outlaw discrimination against people with AIDS. Not the disease but the appeals heard from the most official quarters 'to set aside prejudice and fear in favor of compassion' (the words of the Watkins Report) have become a principal target, suggesting as they do a weakening of this society's power (or willingness) to punish and segregate through judgments about sexual behavior.

More than cancer, but rather like syphilis, AIDS seems to foster ominous fantasies about a disease that is a marker of both individual and social vulnerabilities. The virus invades the body; the disease (or, in the newer version, the fear of the disease) is described as invading the whole society. In late 1986 President Reagan pronounced AIDS to be spreading – 'insidiously' of course – 'through the length and breadth of our society.'* But AIDS, while the pretext for expressing dark intimations about the body politic, has yet to seem credible as a political metaphor for internal enemies, even in France,

---

* Reagan's affirmation through cliché of the frightening reality of a disease of other people contrasts with his more original denial of the reality of his own illness. When asked how he felt after his cancer operation, he declared: 'I didn't have cancer. I had something inside of me that had cancer in it and it was removed.'

where AIDS – in French *le sida* – was quickly added to the store of political invective. Le Pen has dismissed some of his opponents as 'AIDS-ish' (*sidatique*), and the antiliberal polemicist Louis Pauwels said that lycée students on strike last year were suffering from 'mental AIDS' (*sont atteint d'un sida mental*). Neither has AIDS proved of much use as a metaphor for international political evil. True, Jeane Kirkpatrick once couldn't resist comparing international terrorism to AIDS, but such sallies are rare – perhaps because for that purpose the cancer metaphor has proved so fecund.

This doesn't mean that AIDS is not used, preposterously, as a metaphor, but only that AIDS has a metaphoric potential different from that of cancer. When the movie director in Alain Tanner's film *La Vallée Fantôme* (1987) muses, 'Cinema is like a cancer,' and then corrects himself, 'No, it's infectious, it's more like AIDS,' the comparison seems lumberingly self-conscious as well as a decided underuse of AIDS. Not its infectiousness but its characteristic latency offers a more distinctive use of AIDS as a metaphor. Thus, the Palestinian Israeli writer Anton Shammas in the Jerusalem weekly *Kol Ha'ir*, in a fit of medical, sexual, and political fantasy, recently described Israel's Declaration of Independence of 1948 as

the AIDS of 'the Jewish State in the Land of Israel,' whose long incubation has produced Gush Emunim and ... [Rabbi Meir] Kahane. That is where it all began, and that is where it all will end. AIDS, I am sorry to say, despite my sympathy for homosexuals, affects mainly monoerotics, and a mononational Jewish State contains by definition the seeds of its own destruction: the collapse of the political immune system that we call democracy ... Rock Hudson, who once was as beautiful as a Palmachnik, now lies dying long after the dissolution of the Palmach. The State of Israel (for Jews, of course) was indeed once beautiful ...

And even more promising than its connection with latency is the potential of AIDS as a metaphor for contamination and mutation. Cancer is still common as a metaphor for what is feared or deplored, even if the illness is less dreaded than before. If AIDS can eventually be drafted for comparable use, it will be because AIDS is not only invasive (a trait it shares with cancer) or even because it is infectious, but because of the specific imagery that surrounds viruses.

Virology supplies a new set of medical metaphors independent of AIDS which nevertheless reinforce the AIDS mythology. It was years before AIDS that William Burroughs oracularly declared, and Laurie Anderson echoed, 'Language is a virus.' And the viral explanation is invoked more and more often. Until recently, most of the infections recognized as viral were ones, like rabies and influenza, that have very rapid effects. But the category of slow-acting viral infections is growing. Many progressive and invariably fatal disorders of the cental nervous system and some degenerative diseases of the brain that can appear in old age, as well as the so-called auto-immune diseases, are now suspected of being, in fact, slow virus diseases. (And evidence continues to accumulate for a viral cause of at least some human cancers.) Notions of conspiracy translate well into metaphors of implacable, insidious, infinitely patient viruses. In contrast to bacteria, which are relatively complex organisms, viruses are described as an extremely primitive form of life. At the same time, their activities are far more complex than those envisaged in the earlier germ models of infection. Viruses are not simply agents of infection, contamination. They transport genetic 'information,' they transform cells. And they themselves, many of them, evolve. While the smallpox virus appears to stay constant for centuries, influenza viruses evolve so rapidly that vaccines need to be modified every year to keep up with changes in the 'surface coat' of the virus.* The virus or, more accurately, viruses thought to cause AIDS are at least as mutable as the influenza viruses. Indeed, 'virus' is now a synonym for change. Linda Ronstadt, recently explaining why she prefers doing Mexican folk music to rock 'n' roll, observed: 'We don't

* The reason that a vaccine is considered the optimal response to viruses has to do with what makes them 'primitive.' Bacteria have many metabolic differences from mammalian cells and can reproduce outside the cells of their host, which makes it possible to find substances that target them specifically. With viruses, which bond with their host cells, it is a much more difficult problem to distinguish viral functions from normal cellular ones. Hence, the main strategy for controlling viral infections has been the development of vaccines, which do not 'attack' a virus directly (as penicillin attacks infectious bacteria) but 'forestall' infection by stimulating the immune system in advance.

have any tradition in contemporary music except change. Mutate, like a virus.'

So far as 'plague' still has a future as a metaphor, it is through the ever more familiar notion of the virus. (Perhaps no disease in the future caused by a bacillus will be considered as plague-like.) Information itself, now inextricably linked to the powers of computers, is threatened by something compared to a virus. Rogue or pirate programs, known as software viruses, are described as paralleling the behavior of biological viruses (which can capture the genetic code of parts of an organism and effect transfers of alien genetic material). These programs, deliberately planted onto a floppy disk meant to be used with the computer or introduced when the computer is communicating over telephone lines or data networks with other computers, copy themselves onto the computer's operating sytem. Like their biological namesakes, they won't produce immediate signs of damage to the computer's memory, which gives the newly 'infected' program time to spread to other computers. Such metaphors drawn from virology, partly stimulated by the omnipresence of talk of AIDS, are turning up everywhere. (The virus that destroyed a considerable amount of data at the student computer center at Lehigh University of Bethlehem, Pennsylvania, in 1987, was given the name PC AIDS. In France, computer specialists already speak of the problem of *le sida informatique*.) And they reinforce the sense of the omnipresence of AIDS.

It is perhaps not surprising that the newest

transforming element in the modern word, computers, should be borrowing metaphors drawn from our newest transforming illness. Nor is it surprising that descriptions of the course of viral infection now often echo the language of the computer age, as when it is said that a virus will normally produce 'new copies of itself.' In addition to the mechanistic descriptions, the way viruses are animistically characterized – as a menace in waiting, as mutable, as furtive, as biologically innovative – reinforces the sense that a disease can be something ingenious, unpredictable, novel. These metaphors are central to ideas about AIDS that distinguish this illness from others that have been regarded as plague-like. For though the fears AIDS represents are old, its status as that unexpected event, an entirely new disease – a new judgment, as it were – adds to the dread.

Chapter Seven

Some will allow no Diseases to be new, others thi .. that
many old ones are ceased; and that such which are esteemed
new, will have but their time: However, the Mercy of
God hath scattered the great heap of Diseases, and not
loaded any one Country with all: some may be new in one
Country which have been old in another. New Discoveries
of the Earth discover new Diseases ... and if Asia, Africa,
and America should bring in their List, Pandoras Box
would swell, and there must be a strange Pathology.

Sir Thomas Browne,
'A Letter to a Friend, Upon Occasion of
the Death of his Intimate Friend'

It is, of course, unlikely that AIDS, first identified in the
early 1980s, is a new disease. Most probably the virus
has been around a long time, and not only in Africa,
though it is only recently (and in Africa) that the disease
has attained epidemic volume. But for general consciousness it *is* a new disease, and for medicine, too: AIDS

157

marks a turning point in current attitudes towards illness and medicine, as well as toward sexuality and toward catastrophe. Medicine had been viewed as an age-old military campaign now nearing its final phase, leading to victory. The emergence of a new epidemic disease, when for several decades it had been confidently assumed that such calamities belonged to the past, has inevitably changed the status of medicine. The advent of AIDS has made it clear that the infectious diseases are far from conquered and their roster far from closed.

Medicine changed mores. Illness is changing them back. Contraception and the assurance by medicine of the easy curability of sexually transmitted diseases (as of almost all infectious diseases) made it possible to regard sex as an adventure without consequences. Now AIDS obliges people to think of sex as having, possibly, the direst consequences: suicide. Or murder. (There was a trial run for the conversion of sexuality to something dangerous in the widely diffused panic about herpes in the United States in the early 1980s – and herpes in most cases is merely awful, erotically disqualifying.) The fear of AIDS imposes on an act whose ideal is an experience of pure presentness (and a creation of the future) a relation to the past to be ignored at one's peril. Sex no longer withdraws its partners, if only for a moment, from the social. It cannot be considered just a coupling; it is a chain, a chain of transmission, from the past. 'So remember when a person has sex, they're not just having it with that partner, they're having it with everybody that partner had it with for the past ten years,' runs an endearingly gender-vague pronouncement made in 1987 by the Secretary of Health and Human Services, Dr. Otis R. Bowen. AIDS reveals all but long-term monogamous sex as promiscuous (therefore dangerous) and also as deviant, for all heterosexual relations are also homosexual ones, once removed.

Fear of sexuality is the new, disease-sponsored register of the universe of fear in which everyone now lives. Cancerphobia taught us the fear of a polluting environment; now we have the fear of polluting people that AIDS anxiety inevitably communicates. Fear of the Communion cup, fear of surgery: fear of contaminated blood, whether Christ's blood or your neighbor's. Life – blood, sexual fluids – is itself the bearer of contamination. These fluids are potentially lethal. Better to abstain. People are storing their own blood for future use. The model of altruistic behavior in our society, giving blood anonymously, has been compromised, since no one can be sure about anonymous blood received. Not only does AIDS have the unhappy effect of reinforcing American moralism about sex; it further strengthens the culture of self-interest, which is much of what is usually praised as 'individualism.' Self-interest now receives an added boost as simple medical prudence.

All rapid epidemics, including those in which there is no suspicion of sexual transmission or any culpabilizing of the ill, give rise to roughly similar practices of avoidance and exclusion. In the influenza pandemic of 1918–19 – influenza is a highly communicable disease, caused by an airborne virus (transmitted via the respiratory system) – people were advised against shaking hands and urged to put handkerchiefs over their mouths when kissing. Police officers were ordered to don gauze masks before entering a house where people had become ill, as many police officers do today when making arrests in the lower depths, since AIDS in the United States has become increasingly a disease of the urban poor, particularly blacks and Hispanics. Many barbers and dentists wore masks and gloves, as dentists and dental hygienists do now. But the great influenza epidemic, which killed twenty million people, was an affair of fifteen months. With a slow-motion epidemic, these same precautions take on a life of their own. They become part of social mores, not a practice adopted for a brief period of emergency, then discarded.

With an epidemic in which there is no immediate prospect of a vaccine, much less of a cure, prevention plays a larger part in consciousness. But campaigns to keep people from getting ill run into many difficulties with diseases that are venereally transmitted. There has always been reluctance in American health campaigns to communicate information about ways of having safer sex. The *US Guide for Schools* issued in late 1987 by the Department of Education virtually refuses to discuss reducing risk and proposes abstinence as the best way of safeguarding against AIDS, recalling lectures given soldiers during World War I that chastity was the only safeguard against syphilis as well as part of their patriotic duty in fighting the Hun.★ Talk of condoms and clean needles is felt to be tantamount to condoning and abetting illicit sex, illegal chemicals. (And to some extent is. Education about how to keep from getting AIDS does imply an acknowledgment of, therefore tolerance of, the ineradicable variousness of expression of sexual feeling.) European societies, less committed to sexual hypocrisy at the level of public edict, are unlikely to urge people to be chaste as a way of warning them to be prudent. 'Be careful. AIDS.' And 'AIDS. Don't die of ignorance.' The specific meaning of these generalities to be seen on billboards and television spots throughout Western Europe for several years is: Use condoms. But there is a larger meaning in all these messages about being careful, not being ignorant, that will facilitate the acceptance of this kind of public service ad here as well. Part of making an event real is just *saying* it, over and over. In this case, to say it over and over is to instill the consciousness of

★ The other side of this refusal to give instructions about practices that would be less risky was the feeling that it was less than manly to submit one's sexual life to the guidelines of safety and prudence. According to Hemingway's fantasy, in *Death in the Afternoon* (1932): 'Syphilis was the disease of the crusaders in the middle ages. It was supposed to be brought to Europe by them, and it is a disease of all people who lead lives in which disregard of consequences dominates. It is an industrial accident, to be expected by all those who lead irregular sexual lives and from their habits of mind would rather take chances than use prophylactics, and it is a to-be-expected end, or rather phase, of the life of all fornicators who continue their careers far enough.'

risk, the necessity of prudence as such, prior to and superseding any specific recommendation.

Of course, between the perennial official hypocrisy and the fashionable libertinism of recent decades there is a vast gap. The view that sexually transmitted diseases are not serious reached its apogee in the 1970s, which was also when many male homosexuals reconstituted themselves as something like an ethnic group, one whose distinctive folkloric custom was sexual voracity, and the institutions of urban homosexual life became a sexual delivery system of unprecedented speed, efficiency, and volume. Fear of AIDS enforces a much more moderate exercise of appetite, and not just among homosexual men. In the United States sexual behavior pre-1981 now seems for the middle class part of a lost age of innocence – innocence in the guise of licentiousness, of course. After two decades of sexual spending, of sexual speculation, of sexual inflation, we are in the early stages of a sexual depression. Looking back on the sexual culture of the 1970s has been compared to looking back on the jazz age from the wrong side of the 1929 crash.

One set of messages of the society we live in is: Consume. Grow. Do what you want. Amuse yourselves. The very working of this economic system, which has bestowed these unprecedented liberties, most cherished in the form of physical mobility and material prosperity, depends on encouraging people to defy limits. Appetite is *supposed* to be immoderate. The ideology of capitalism makes us all into connoisseurs of liberty – of the indefinite expansion of possibility. Virtually every kind of advocacy claims to offer first of all or also some increment of freedom. Not every freedom, to be sure. In rich countries, freedom has come to be identified more and more with 'personal fulfillment' – a freedom enjoyed or practiced alone (or *as* alone). Hence much of recent discourse about the body, reimagined as the instrument with which to enact, increasingly, various programs of self-improvement, of the heightening of powers. Given the imperatives about consumption and the virtually unquestioned value attached to the expression of self, how could sexuality *not* have come to be, for some, a consumer option: an exercise of liberty, of increased mobility, of the pushing back of limits. Hardly an invention of the male homosexual subculture, recreational, risk-free sexuality is an inevitable reinvention of the culture of capitalism, and was guaranteed by medicine as well. The advent of AIDS seems to have changed all that, irrevocably.

AIDS magnifies the force of the quite different yet complementary messages increasingly heard by people in this society accustomed to being able to provide pleasures for themselves, more and more of whom are drawn to programs of self-management and self-discipline (diet, exercise). Watch your appetites. Take care of yourself. Don't let yourself go. Limits have long been set on the indulgence of certain appetites in the name of health or of the creation of an ideal physical appearance – voluntary limits, an exercise of freedom. The catastrophe of AIDS suggests the immediate *necessity* of limitation, of constraint for the body and for to a very real danger. It also expresses a positive desire, the desire for stricter limits in the conduct of personal life. There is a broad tendency in our culture, an end-of-an-era feeling, that AIDS is reinforcing; an exhaustion, for many, of purely secular ideals – ideals that seemed to encourage libertinism or at least not provide any coherent inhibition against it – in which the response to AIDS finds its place. The behavior AIDS is stimulating is part of a larger grateful return to what is perceived as 'conventions,' like the return to figure and landscape, tonality and melody, plot and character, and other much vaunted repudiations of difficult modernism in the arts. The reduction in the imperative of promiscuity in the middle class, a growth of the ideal of monogamy, of a prudent sexual life, is as marked in, say, Stockholm, with its tiny number of AIDS cases, as it is in New York, where the disease can accurately be called of epidemic proportions. The response to AIDS, while in part perfectly rational, amplifies a widespread questioning that had been rising in intensity throughout the 1970s of many of the ideals (and risks) of enlightened modernity; and the new sexual realism goes with the rediscovery of the joys of tonal music, Bouguereau, a career in investment banking, and church weddings.

The mounting panic about the risks of recreational and commercialized sexuality is unlikely to diminish the attractions of other kinds of appetites: boutiques are expected to fill the building in Hamburg until recently occupied by the Eros Center. Sexual exchanges are to be carried out only after forethought. Routine consumption of drugs that boosted energies for mental work and for palaver (what also rose throughout the 1970s was bourgeois cocaine use) has played its part in preparing for the neo-celibacy and waning of sexual spontaneity common among the educated in this decade. Machines supply new, popular ways of inspiring desire and keeping it safe, as mental as possible: the commercially organized lechery by telephone (and in France by 'Minitel') that offers a version of anonymous promiscuous sex without the exchange of fluids. And strictures about contact now have their place in the computer world as well. Computer users are advised to regard each new piece of software as a 'potential carrier' of a virus. 'Never put a disk in your computer without verifying its source.' The so-called vaccine programs being marketed are said to offer some protection; but the only sure way to curb the threat of computer viruses, experts agree, is not to share programs and data. The culture of consumption may actually be stimulated by the warnings to consumers of all kinds of goods and services to be more cautious, more selfish. For these anxieties will require the further replication of goods and services.

Chapter Eight

Epidemics of particularly dreaded illnesses always pro-
voke an outcry against leniency or tolerance — now
identified as laxity, weakness, disorder, corruption: un-
healthiness. Demands are made to subject people to
'tests,' to isolate the ill and those suspected of being ill or
of transmitting illness, and to erect barriers against the
real or imaginary contamination of foreigners. Societies
already administered as garrisons, like China (with a tiny
number of detected cases) and Cuba (with a significant
number of the already ill), are responding more rapidly
and peremptorily. AIDS is everyone's Trojan horse: six
months before the 1988 Olympics the South Korean
government announced that it would be distributing
free condoms to all foreign participants. 'This is a totally
foreign disease, and the only way to stop its spread is to
stop sexual contacts between Indians and foreigners,'
declared the director general of the Indian government's
Council for Medical Research, thereby avowing the total

defenselessness of a population nearing a billion for which there are presently *no* trained hospital staff members or treatment centers anywhere specializing in the disease. His proposal for a sexual ban, to be enforced by fines and prison terms, is no less impractical as a means of curbing sexually transmitted diseases than the more commonly made proposals for quarantine – that is, for detention. The incarceration in detention camps surrounded by barbed wire during World War I of some thirty thousand American women, prostitutes and women suspected of being prostitutes, for the avowed purpose of controlling syphilis among army recruits, caused no drop in the military's rate of infection – just as incarceration during World War II of tens of thousands of Americans of Japanese ancestry as potential traitors and spies probably did not foil a single act of espionage or sabotage. That does not mean that comparable proposals for AIDS will not be made, or will not find support, and not only by the predictable people. If the medical establishment has been on the whole a bulwark of sanity and rationality so far, refusing even to envisage programs of quarantine and detention, it may be in part because the dimensions of the crisis still seem limited and the evolution of the disease unclear.

Uncertainty about how much the disease will spread – how soon and to whom – remains at the center of public discourse about AIDS. Will it, as it spreads around the world, remain restricted, largely, to marginal populations: to the so-called risk groups and then to large sections of the urban poor? Or will it eventually become the classic pandemic affecting entire regions? Both views are in fact being held simultaneously. A wave of statements and articles affirming that AIDS threatens everybody is followed by another wave of articles asserting that it is a disease of 'them,' not 'us.' At the beginning of 1987, the US Secretary of Health and Human Services predicted that the worldwide AIDS epidemic would eventually make the Black Death – the greatest epidemic ever recorded, which wiped out between a third and a half of the population of Europe – seem 'pale by comparison.' At the end of the year he said: 'This is not a massive, widely spreading epidemic among heterosexuals as so many people fear.' Even more striking than the cyclical character of public discourse about AIDS is the readiness of so many to envisage the most far-reaching of catastrophes.

Reassurances are multiplying in the United States and Western Europe that 'the general population' is safe. But 'the general population' may be as much a code phrase for whites as it is for heterosexuals. Everyone knows that blacks are getting AIDS in disproportionate numbers, as there is a disproportionate number of blacks in the armed forces and a vastly disproportionate number in prisons. 'The AIDS virus is an equal-opportunity destroyer' was the slogan of a recent fund-raising campaign by the American Foundation for AIDS Research. Punning on 'equal-opportunity employer,' the phrase subliminally reaffirms what it means to deny: that AIDS is an illness that in this part of the world afflicts minorities, racial and sexual. And about the staggering prediction made recently by the World Health Organization that, barring improbably rapid progress in the development of a vaccine, there will be ten to twenty times more AIDS cases in the next five years than there were in the last five, it is assumed that most of these millions will be Africans.

AIDS quickly became a global event – discussed not only in New York, Paris, Rio, Kinshasa but also in Helsinki, Buenos Aires, Beijing, and Singapore – when it was far from the leading cause of death in Africa, much less in the world. There are famous diseases, as there are famous countries, and these are not necessarily the ones with the biggest populations. AIDS did not become so famous just because it afflicts whites too, as some Africans bitterly assert. But it is certainly true that were AIDS only an African disease, however many millions were dying, few outside of Africa would be concerned with it. It would be one of those 'natural' events, like famines, which periodically ravage poor, overpopulated countries and about which people in rich countries feel quite helpless. Because it is a world event – that is, because it affects the West – it is regarded as not just a natural disaster. It is filled with historical meaning. (Part of the self-definition of Europe and neo-European countries is that it, the First World, is where major calamities are history-making, transformative, while in poor, African or Asian countries they are part of a cycle, and therefore something like an aspect of nature.) Nor has AIDS become so publicized because, as some have suggested, in rich countries the illness first afflicted a group of people who were all men, almost all white, many of them educated, articulate, and knowledgeable about how to lobby and organize for public attention and resources devoted to the disease. AIDS occupies such a large part in our awareness because of what it has been taken to represent. It seems the very model of all the catastrophes privileged populations feel await them.

What biologists and public health officials predict is something far worse than can be imagined or than society (and the economy) can tolerate. No responsible official holds out the slightest hope that the African economies and health services can cope with the spread of the disease predicted for the near future, while every day one can read the direst estimates of the cost of AIDS to the country that has reported the largest number of cases, the United States. Astonishingly large sums of money are cited as the cost of providing minimum care to people who will be ill in the next few years. (This is assuming that the reassurances to 'the general population' are justified, an assumption much disputed within the medical community.) Talk in the United States, and not only in the United States, is of a national emergency, 'possibly our nation's survival.' An editorialist at *The New York Times* intoned last year: 'We all know the truth, every one of us. We live in a time of plague such as has never been visited on our nation. We can pretend it does not exist, or exists for those others, and carry on as if we do not know . . .' And one French poster shows a giant UFO-like black mass hovering over and darkening with spidery rays most of the familiar hexagon shape of the country lying below. Above the image is written: 'It depends on each of us to erase that shadow' (*Il dépend de chacun de nous d'effacer cette ombre*). And underneath: 'France doesn't want to die of AIDS' (*La France ne veut pas mourir du sida*). Such token appeals for mass mobilization to confront an unprecedented menace appear, at frequent intervals, in every mass society. It is also typical of a modern society that the demand for mobilization be kept very general and the reality of the response fall well short of what seems to be demanded to meet the challenge of the nation-endangering menace. This sort of rhetoric has a life of its own: it serves some purpose if it simply keeps in circulation an ideal of unifying communal practice that is precisely contradicted by the pursuit of accumulation and isolating entertainments enjoined on the citizens of a modern mass society.

The survival of the nation, of civilized society, of the world itself is said to be at stake – claims that are a familiar part of building a case for repression. (An emergency requires 'drastic measures,' et cetera.) The end-of-the-world rhetoric that AIDS has evoked does inevitably build such a case. But it also does something else. It offers a stoic, finally numbing contemplation of catastrophe. The eminent Harvard historian of science Stephen Jay Gould has declared that the AIDS pandemic may rank with nuclear weaponry 'as the greatest danger of our era.' But even if it kills as much as a quarter of the human race – a prospect Gould considers possible –

'there will still be plenty of us left and we can start again.' Scornful of the jeremiads of the moralists, a rational and humane scientist proposes the minimum consolation: an apocalypse that doesn't have any meaning. AIDS is a 'natural phenomenon,' not an event 'with a moral meaning,' Gould points out; 'there is no message in its spread.' Of course, it is monstrous to attribute meaning, in the sense of moral judgment, to the spread of an infectious disease. But perhaps it is only a little less monstrous to be invited to contemplate death on this horrendous scale with equanimity.

Much of the well-intentioned public discourse in our time expresses a desire to be candid about one or another of the various dangers which might be leading to all-out catastrophe. And now there is one more. To the death of oceans and lakes and forests, the unchecked growth of populations in the poor parts of the world, nuclear accidents like Chernobyl, the puncturing and depletion of the ozone layer, the perennial threat of nuclear confrontation between the superpowers or nuclear attack by one of the rogue states not under superpower control – to all these, now add AIDS. In the countdown to a millennium, a rise in apocalyptic thinking may be inevitable. Still, the amplitude of the fantasies of doom that AIDS has inspired can't be explained by the calendar alone, or even by the very real danger the illness represents. There is also the need for an apocalyptic scenario that is specific to 'Western' society, and perhaps even more so to the United States. (America, as someone has said, is a nation with the soul of a church – an evangelical church prone to announcing radical endings and brand-new beginnings.) The taste for worst-case scenarios reflects the need to master fear of what is felt to be uncontrollable. It also expresses an imaginative complicity with disaster. The sense of cultural distress or failure gives rise to the desire for a clean sweep, a tabula rasa. No one wants a plague, of course. But, yes, it would be a chance to begin again. And beginning again – that is very modern, very American, too.

AIDS may be extending the propensity for becoming inured to vistas of global annihilation which the stocking and brandishing of nuclear arms has already promoted. With the inflation of apocalyptic rhetoric has come the increasing unreality of the apocalypse. A permanent modern scenario: apocalypse looms ... and it doesn't occur. And it still looms. We seem to be in the throes of one of the modern kinds of apocalypse. There is the one that's not happening, whose outcome remains in suspense: the missiles circling the earth above our heads, with a nuclear payload that could destroy all life many times over, that haven't (so far) gone off. And there are ones that are happening, and yet seem not to have (so far) the most feared consequences – like the astronomical Third World debt, like overpopulation, like ecological blight; or that happen and then (we are told) didn't happen – like the October 1987 stock market collapse, which was a 'crash,' like the one in October 1929, and was not. Apocalypse is now a long-running serial: not 'Apocalypse Now' but 'Apocalypse From Now On.' Apocalypse has become an event that is happening and not happening. It may be that some of the most feared events, like those involving the irreparable ruin of the environment, have already happened. But we don't know it yet, because the standards have changed. Or because we do not have the right indices for measuring the catastrophe. Or simply because this is a catastrophe in slow motion. (Or *feels* as if it is in slow motion, because we know about it, can anticipate it; and now have to wait for it to happen, to catch up with what we think we know.)

Modern life accustoms us to live with the intermittent awareness of monstrous, unthinkable – but, we are told, quite probable – disasters. Every major event is haunted, and not only by its representation as an image (an old doubling of reality now, which began in 1839, with the invention of the camera). Besides the photographic or electronic simulation of events, there is also the calculation of their eventual outcome. Reality has bifurcated, into the real thing and an alternative version of it, twice over. There is the event and its image. And there is the event and its projection. But as real events often seem to have no more reality for people than images, and to need the confirmation of their images, so our reaction to events in the present seeks confirmation in a mental outline, with appropriate computations, of the event in its projected, ultimate form.

Future-mindedness is as much the distinctive mental habit, and intellectual corruption, of this century as the history-mindedness that, as Nietzsche pointed out, transformed thinking in the nineteenth century. Being able to estimate how matters will evolve into the future is an inevitable byproduct of a more sophisticated (quantifiable, testable) understanding of process, social as well as scientific. The ability to project events with some accuracy into the future enlarged what power consisted of, because it was a vast new source of instructions about how to deal with the present. But in fact the look into the future, which was once tied to a vision of linear progress, has, with more knowledge at our disposal than anyone could have dreamed, turned into a vision of disaster. Every process is a prospect, and invites a prediction bolstered by statistics. Say: the number now . . . in three years, in five years, in ten years; and, of course, at the end of the century. Anything in history or nature that can be described as changing steadily can be seen as heading toward catastrophe. (Either the too little and becoming less: waning, decline, entropy. Or the too much, ever more than we can handle or absorb: uncontrollable growth.) Most of what experts pronounce about the future contributes to this new double sense of reality – beyond the doubleness to which we are already accustomed by the comprehensive duplication of everything in images. There is what is happening now. And there is what it portends: the imminent, but not yet actual, and not really graspable, disaster.

Two kinds of disaster, actually. And a gap between them, in which the imagination flounders. The difference between the epidemic we have and the pandemic that we are promised (by current statistical extrapolations) feels like the difference between the wars we have, so-called limited wars, and the unimaginably more terrible ones we could have, the latter (with all the appurtenances of science fiction) being the sort of activity people are addicted to staging for fun, as electronic games. For beyond the real epidemic with its inexorably mounting death toll (statistics are issued by national and international health organizations every week, every month) is a qualitatively different, much greater disaster which we think both will and will not take place. Nothing is changed when the most appalling estimates are revised downward, temporarily, which is an occasional feature of the display of speculative statistics disseminated by health bureaucrats and journalists. Like the demographic predictions, which are probably just as accurate, the big news is usually bad.

A proliferation of reports or projections of unreal (that is, ungraspable) doomsday eventualities tends to produce a variety of reality-denying responses. Thus, in most discussions of nuclear warfare, being rational (the self-description of experts) means not acknowledging the human reality, while taking in emotionally even a small part of what is at stake for human beings (the province of those who regard themselves as the menaced) means insisting on unrealistic demands for the rapid dismantling of the peril. This split of public attitude, into the inhuman and the all-too-human, is much less stark with AIDS. Experts denounce the stereotypes attached to people with AIDS and to the continent where it is presumed to have originated, emphasizing that the disease belongs to much wider populations than the groups initially at risk, and to the whole world, not just to Africa.* For while AIDS has turned out, not surprisingly, to be one of the most meaning-laden of diseases, along with leprosy and syphilis, clearly there are checks on the impulse to stigmatize people with the disease. The way in which the illness is such a perfect repository for people's most general fears about the future to some extent renders irrelevant the predictable efforts to pin the disease on a deviant group or a dark continent.

Like the effects of industrial pollution and the new system of global financial markets, the AIDS crisis is evidence of a world in which nothing important is regional, local, limited; in which everything that can circulate does, and every problem is, or is destined to become,

* 'AIDS cannot be stopped in any country unless it is stopped in all countries,' declared the retiring head of the World Health Organization in Geneva, Dr. Halfdan Mahler, at the Fourth International Conference on AIDS (Stockholm, June 1988), where the global character of the AIDS crisis was a leading theme. 'This epidemic is worldwide and is sparing no continent,' said Dr. Willy Rozenbaum, a French AIDS specialist. 'It cannot be mastered in the West unless it is overcome everywhere.' In contrast to the rhetoric of global responsibility, a specialty of the international conferences, is the view, increasingly heard, in which AIDS is regarded as a kind of Darwinian test of a society's aptitude for survival, which may require writing off those countries that can't defend themselves. A German AIDS specialist, Dr. Eike Brigitte Helm, has declared that it 'can already be seen that in a number of parts of the world AIDS will drastically change the population structure. Particularly in Africa and Latin America. A society that is not able, somehow or other, to prevent the spread of AIDS has very poor prospects for the future.'

worldwide. Goods circulate (including images and sounds and documents, which circulate fastest of all, electronically). Garbage circulates: the poisonous industrial wastes of St. Etienne, Hannover, Mestre, and Bristol are being dumped in the coastal towns of West Africa. People circulate, in greater numbers than ever. And diseases. From the untrammeled intercontinental air travel for pleasure and business of the privileged to the unprecedented migrations of the underprivileged from villages to cities and, legally and illegally, from country to country – all this physical mobility and interconnectedness (with its consequent dissolving of old taboos, social and sexual) is as vital to the maximum functioning of the advanced, or world, capitalist economy as is the easy transmissibility of goods and images and financial instruments. But now that heightened, modern interconnectedness in space, which is not only personal but social, structural, is the bearer of a health menace sometimes described as a threat to the species itself; and the fear of AIDS is of a piece with attention to other unfolding disasters that are the byproducts of advanced society, particularly those illustrating the degradation of the environment on a world scale. AIDS is one of the dystopian harbingers of the global village, that future which is already here and always before us, which no one knows how to refuse.

That even an apocalypse can be made to seem part of the ordinary horizon of expectation constitutes an unparalleled violence that is being done to our sense of reality, to our humanity. But it is highly desirable for a specific dreaded illness to come to seem ordinary. Even the disease most fraught with meaning can become just an illness. It has happened with leprosy, though some ten million people in the world, easy to ignore since almost all live in Africa and the Indian subcontinent, have what is now called, as part of its wholesome de-dramatization, Hansen's disease (after the Norwegian physician who, over a century ago, discovered the bacillus). It is bound to happen with AIDS, when the illness is much better understood and, above all, treatable. For the time being, much in the way of individual experience and social policy depends on the struggle for rhetorical ownership of the illness: how it is possessed, assimilated in argument and in cliché. The age-old, seemingly inexorable process whereby diseases acquire meanings (by coming to stand for the deepest fears) and inflict stigma is always worth challenging, and it does seem to have more limited credibility in the modern world, among people willing to be modern – the process is under surveillance now. With this illness, one that elicits so much guilt and shame, the effort to detach it from these meanings, these metaphors, seems particularly liberating, even consoling. But the metaphors cannot be distanced just by abstaining from them. They have to be exposed, criticized, belabored, used up.

Not all metaphors applied to illnesses and their treatment are equally unsavory and distorting. The one I am most eager to see retired – more than ever since the emergence of AIDS – is the military metaphor. Its converse, the medical model of the public weal, is probably more dangerous and far-reaching in its consequences, since it not only provides a persuasive justification for authoritarian rule but implicitly suggests the necessity of state-sponsored repression and violence (the equivalent of surgical removal or chemical control of the offending or 'unhealthy' parts of the body politic). But the effect of the military imagery on thinking about sickness and health is far from inconsequential. It over-mobilizes, it overdescribes, and it powerfully contributes to the excommunicating and stigmatizing of the ill.

No, it is not desirable for medicine, any more than for war, to be 'total.' Neither is the crisis created by AIDS a 'total' anything. We are not being invaded. The body is not a battlefield. The ill are neither unavoidable casualties nor the enemy. We – medicine, society – are not authorized to fight back by any means whatever . . . About that metaphor, the military one, I would say, if I may paraphrase Lucretius: Give it back to the war-makers.

UNDER THE SIGN OF SATURN

Susan Sontag

Susan Sontag's third essay collection brings together her most important critical writing from 1972 to 1980. In these provocative and hugely influential works she explores some of the most controversial artists and thinkers of our time, including her now-famous polemic against Hitler's favourite film-maker, Leni Riefenstahl, and the cult of fascist art, as well as a dazzling analysis of Hans-Jürgen Syberberg's *Hitler: a Film from Germany*. There are also highly personal and powerful explorations of death, art, language, history, the imagination and writing itself.

'After this feast, I am eager for her thoughts on anything' *Chicago Sun Times*

IN AMERICA

Susan Sontag

The story of *In America* is inspired by the emigration to America in 1876 of Helena Modrzejewska, Poland's most celebrated actress, accompanied by her husband, Count Karol Chlapowski, her fifteen-year-old son, Rudolf, the young journalist and future author of *Quo Vadis*, Henryk Sienkiewicz, and a few friends; their brief sojourn in Anaheim, California; and Modrzejewska's subsequent triumphant career on the American stage under the name Helena Modjeska.

'A tour de force. . . . A magical accomplishment by an alchemist of ideas and words, images and truth' Michael Pakenham, *The Baltimore Sun*

CHERNOBYL PRAYER

Svetlana Alexievich

On 26 April 1986 the worst nuclear reactor accident in history occured in Chernobyl and contaminated as much as three quarters of Europe. While the official Soviet narrative downplayed the accident's impact, Svetlana Alexievich wanted to know how people understood it. She recorded hundreds of interviews with workers at the nuclear plant, refugees and resettlers, scientists and bureaucrats, crafting their monologues into a stunning oral history of the nuclear disaster. What their stories reveal is the fear, anger and uncertainty with which they still live but also a dark humour and desire to see the beauty of everyday life, including that of Chernobyl's new landscape. A chronicle of the past and a warning for our nuclear future, *Chernobyl Prayer* is a haunting masterpiece.

'A searing mix of eloquence and wordlessness . . . From her interviewees' monologues she creates history that the reader, at whatever distance from the events, can actually touch' Julian Evans, *The Telegraph*

NOTES OF A NATIVE SON

James Baldwin

Written during the 1940s and early 1950s, when Baldwin was only in his twenties, the essays collected in *Notes of a Native Son* capture a view of black life and black thought at the dawn of the civil rights movement. Writing as an artist, activist and social critic, Baldwin probes the complex condition of being black in America – from life in Harlem, to the protest novel, movies, and the experience of African Americans abroad – and many of his observations have proven almost prophetic.

This book inaugurated Baldwin as one of the leading interpreters of the dramatic social changes erupting in the United States in the twentieth century and it is the book that established Baldwin's voice as a social critic. In an age of Black Lives Matter, Baldwin's essays are as powerful today as when they were first written.

'Cemented his reputation as a cultural seer … *Notes of a Native Son* endures as his defining work, and his greatest' *Time*